Quest
for the Killers

Quest
for the Killers

June Goodfield

A *Pro Scientia Viva* Title

B

Birkhäuser

Boston • Basel • Stuttgart

June Goodfield
Quest for the Killers

Companion volume to the PBS Television Series

U.K. edition, titled *From the Face of the Earth,* published by André Deutsch Ltd., 105 Great Russell Street, London WC1B 3LJ.

First printing, August 1985

Library of Congress Cataloging-in-Publication Data

Goodfield, G. J. (G. June), 1927 –
  Quest for the killers.

  "A Pro scientia viva title."
  1. Medicine – Research – Developing countries.
2. Medical scientists – Developing countries.
3. Medicine, Preventive – Developing countries.
I. Title.
R854.D44G66 1985   614.4'09172'4   85-13385
ISBN 0-8176-3313-8

CIP-Kurztitelaufnahme der Deutschen Bibliothek

Goodfield, June:
Quest for the killers / June Goodfield. – Boston;
Basel ; Stuttgart : Birkhäuser, 1985.
  (A Pro Scientia Viva Title)
  ISBN 3-7643-3313-8 (Stuttgart . . .)
  ISBN 0-8176-3313-8 (Boston . . .)

© 1985, by June Goodfield

Published simultaneously in Canada

ISBN 0-8176-3313-8
   3-7643-3313-8

Manufactured in the United States of America

For
Frances Lindley

The color illustrations in this book
were made possible by a grant from
Squibb Corporation.

The author and publisher would like
to thank

D. Carleton Gajdusek
Compix
Axel Poignant
Michael Johnstone
Institute for Basic Research in
    Developmental Disabilities,
    Staten Island, N.Y.
Donna Harley
Merck Institute for Therapeutic Research
Michael Houldey
The Rockefeller Foundation
Pfizer
David Collison
Alan Patient

for granting permission to reproduce
the illustrations in this book.

Contents

*Concern for man himself and his fate
must always form the chief interest of all technical
endeavors . . . never forget this, in the midst of
your diagrams and equations.*

Albert Einstein
Science and Values

Preface

The five stories in this book are tales about human beings and the human condition in which they find themselves. They are stories of scientists – but not of white-coated laboratory figures, happy to leave to others the practical application of their discoveries. In the circumstances I recount, the scientists were brought face to face, sometimes in dramatic confrontations, with the very people whose problems their work might help solve. As I came to realize, there now exists an international network of unusual scientists whose members are concerned individuals, determined that their scientific work should help alleviate the human condition.

This book was conceived as an account of some exciting episodes in contemporary biomedicine. But during the four years it took to complete, several other themes emerged. First, each story illustrates aspects of the relation between Western science and technology and those major health problems which are often of dreadful significance for the Third World. In this relation the fruits of Western research are not simply applied to global health problems. Rather the relation is reciprocal, for scientific research, whether prompted by the medical problems of the Third World or actually conducted there, is yielding vital clues to many fundamental aspects of human biology, as well as pointing toward possible therapies for the serious diseases of Western society, such as cancer or the dementias of old age.

After I had written the first draft a second theme emerged. For I realized that, given a new chronological order, the stories in this book trace the inescapable path that must be traveled from the moment doctors identify a new disease and then pinpoint its cause (Chapter 1), to the moment of ultimate medical triumph, when the disease is eradicated or completely controlled (Chapter 5). One dream of man was encapsulated by Pasteur when he spoke of "eradicating disease from the face of the earth." Though we have only once achieved such success, there is no reason why we should not do so again, even granted that the elimination of all diseases is impossible. But between the two extremes of ignorance and triumph, several other steps lie along the path of our quest. Once the cause of a disease has been identified, a remedy must be devised and a clinical trial mounted to test it (Chapter 2). Where more than one method proves to be practical and efficacious, criteria must be developed for determining which is most suitable, or beneficial, or cost-effective, and these criteria are not always synonymous (Chapter 3). In Chapter 4 we are led from science to its application, from the world of the mind and the laboratory experiment to the real world of human beings, where factors totally extraneous to science – human aspirations, venalities, politics, and other social considerations – come to impinge, factors that finally determine whether any particular medical solution will be applied. Only once in the history of the world did all elements, scientific and human, come together – in the global eradication of smallpox (Chapter 5).

Given the need to weave scientific, political, and human themes, research for this book afforded me an unrivaled opportunity to travel to a variety of fascinating locations and work among people I had never before met, in cultures far remote from my own. The combination of scientific detective work and remarkable locations made these stories excellent candidates for a television series. This has now been completed and the making of the five films has greatly influenced the way the book developed.

My debts are enormous, and some are very obvious. The greatest is undoubtedly to the scientists who worked with me on and off for four years. In a variety of places and encounters, we met, parted, met again several times over, and finally worked together in the creative environment of a film location. Throughout all this time, with understanding for what I was trying to do, they gave unstintingly of their time and their knowledge. They supported and sustained me both directly and by their obvious commitment to the project, and this was equally true of all members of the television production team. Topping all of them by several years, some by at least twenty, there is no doubt that if anybody qualified for the role of grandmother, I did. So I suspect that, in later years, as I recollect these wonderful times, I shall come to resemble the aged Connie in John le Carré's *Tinker, Tailor, Soldier, Spy* who, in a haze of nostalgia induced in her case by equal parts of emotion and alcohol, would regularly murmur "Oh my lovely boys." But in this case there are girls too.

I owe a great deal to many other people besides, and after reading Chapter 2 it will be quite apparent why Mrs. Maya Szmuness and Dr. Aaron Kellner count among these. There were also those who made the project possible, those who supported me and helped throughout, and, finally, some very special people indeed.

It was the Division of Health Sciences and the Division of Humanities at the Rockefeller Foundation who underwrote the research for this book and therefore, indirectly, the research for the television series. The Foundation has had a long and magnificent tradition supporting research into global health problems and its Director of Health Sciences, Dr. Kenneth Warren, has been both a stalwart support and a highly informed and exacting critic. In thanking him for his crucial help, I must also thank Dr. James Hirsch, President of the Josiah Macy Foundation, who, when I first raised the idea, said, "You've got to come and talk to Ken Warren," and arranged the meeting. I am also grateful to Dr. Joshua Lederberg, President of the Rockefeller University, not only for the hospitality of his famous institution for six years, but also for enormous encouragement throughout the project.

Tom Meikle, Dean of Cornell University Medical School, Vera Rubin, Aleck Bearn, Pat Garvey, Frances McGregor, Wylie Merritt, John Mather were of enormous help, and my gratitude is deep. I must mention especially Peter McGhee, John Carver, and Karl Rosenberger, all of WGBH-TV Boston, who worked tremendously hard for the series and sweetly put up with my unfortunate habit of telephoning very early in the morning. Though they were undoubtedly cursing me under their breath, they always were wonderfully polite and enormously helpful. I am grateful too, to Michael Peacock and Dr. Robert Reid of Video Arts Television for sensing the merit in these stories and for their commitment to the production. Without the help of Michael Johnstone, who researched two of these films, Chapter 1 and Chapter 4 of this book would be but pale shadows of what they presently are. He brought a meticulous intelligence and great energy to unraveling their complicated scientific themes.

Christine Gadd and her friends and colleagues at British Airways made the miles I flew as painless as they could. Hilary Rubinstein and Anne Borchardt, who have been my agents on each side of the Atlantic for many years, gave their usual effective, warm, and critical support. Ann Wickens and Joy Beattie helped type various drafts of this book, with patience and humor throughout; Muriel Haynes-Adams, whose apartment in New York provides me with a haven every time I arrive, did stalwart work in rereading and criticizing successive drafts. I would regularly turn up from somewhere, place yet another pile of paper on her table, whereupon with apparent pleasure she would get to work. I am very grateful to her for all her help. Lore Henlein, whose *Pro Scientia Viva* imprint is on the title page, and Klaus Peters of Birkhäuser Boston, worked miracles on editing and production to get this book through press in time. Equally I must express deep gratitude to Jo Elwyn-Jones, who has been associated with this project since its inception. She helped conceptualize the series and acted as a liaison between me and a world with which I was then unfamiliar. As the permanent member of the WGBH staff attached to the production in London, she contributed greatly toward the finished project.

But I am deeply grateful to three people in particular. It was a wonderful experience to work with a professional of such high caliber as Michael Latham, Executive Producer of the series. He focused my thoughts, tightened my arguments, molded the films, and drew out aspects of the stories I never realized existed, and made my first venture into television a delight.

Denise McClean played a critical and seminal role in the entire venture. As my assistant for three and a half years she worked on every aspect of the project, whether research or fund-raising, manuscript work or critical comment. I could not have survived without her.

Finally I must mention Frances Lindley, to whom this book is dedicated with love and gratitude. Her perceptive and invaluable comments, her critical belief in what I was trying to achieve were invaluable. Most important, she never once allowed me to forget that a chapter in a book and a film on television are two quite different things, and, no matter how exalted or exhausted I was, I should never be tempted to dissolve the distinction.

New York and *Alfriston*   June Goodfield

Quest
for the Killers

I
The Kuru Mystery

*Faith is the substance of things hoped for,
the evidence of things not seen.*

Paul's Epistle to the Hebrews, 11,1

Even though most unexplored areas of the world opened up rapidly after the end of World War II, the Eastern Highlands of Papua New Guinea remained remote and isolated. Few outsiders had ever penetrated the territory. Most who did found the experience unnerving, for they encountered "tribes"* of indigenous people living as in the Stone Age, with fearsome reputations as savage warriors and cannibals. Yet, one night in May 1957, a few members of one group, the Fore, were calmly watching a white man perform an autopsy on a young boy who had died shortly after midnight. By the time the body was laid on a rough table in a native hut, it was two o'clock in the morning. A fierce tropical storm was raging, so the crash of thunder, the hiss of rain, the shriek of wind, and the restless shadows thrown by a swinging lantern provided a macabre counterpoint to the cuts into the corpse. Using just a simple carving knife and a saw, and helped by a local *dokta boi* (native medical assistant), the stranger carefully slit into the scalp and then into the skull. With bare hands he lifted the brain from its bony shelter and sliced it into thin sections – not an easy task, the brain still being soft. Samples of other tissues were placed in bottles of formaldehyde and saline, already prepared for shipment. Such was the tension that the doctor worried: perhaps he had wrongly labeled abdominal wall, or lung, or spleen.

As the crowing of the cock announced the impending dawn, the man finished the task and the body was borne homeward by the mourning mother. She carried besides rewards of axes, salt, and *lap-lap,*† gifts that were both fascinating and diverting, for she had been long resigned to the death itself. In her resignation lay clues as to why this "dastardly deed" was permitted and why, indeed, the Fore people were willing to help the

---

* In the New Guinea Highlands there were no true "tribes," but rather many distinct cultural and linguistic groups in scattered villages or hamlets, not linked by "tribal" organization.

† a wrap-around cloth skirt worn by men

stranger. This boy was the latest victim of a terrible affliction that was decimating the Fore. Sorcerers, they said, had cursed them with a wasting, shaking, demonic disease, which was relentlessly picking off its victims one by one. Soon the entire Fore people would be extinct. Perhaps this white man might bring a cure, as others had earlier, with penicillin injections for yaws. Though he yearned to do just that, the stranger knew that first he would need to collect brains from as many victims as he could. He was convinced that within the brain lay clues not only to the mystery of the Fore's strange disease, but to the degenerative diseases of the nervous system found in Western society. This was why he was in the Fore's territory.

The spine of Papua New Guinea is formed by long chains of mountains that climb to fifteen thousand feet, its precipitous slopes and vertical cliffs dissected by steep mountain torrents always in full spate. The Eastern Highlands are covered by the jungle greens of the rain forest on their lower, misty reaches, but between the high peaks rising two miles above sea level are open areas of grassland. The relentless flow of forest and grassland is punctuated by groups of houses, sometimes spread straight along a ridge or arranged in horseshoe shape in the grasslands. Raging rivers separate the valleys and, in 1957, only a few dirt tracks, passable by a Land Rover, linked the Kainantu administrative center and airstrip; no road yet connected with the coast. To reach the Fore had involved days of exhausted effort, hacking through the jungle, sweating along the small tracks known only to the local people, plagued by nettles and razor-sharp grasses, pestered by bees, mosquitoes, snakes, and leeches.

So isolated were the hamlets that the Highland people spoke dozens of completely different languages and one tribe could communicate with another only through those few of their number who had become bilingual through marriage exchanges or adoptions. The first metal axe had come to the country less than twenty years before; it would take twenty years more before the last language group would come into contact with Western civilization.

For centuries then the lives of the Fore had been circumscribed and all outside contacts severely impeded. Their population density was always small – about thirty-five persons per square mile – and by 1957 the fourteen thousand Fore were spread over four hundred square miles.

The Australians had established observation posts in the highlands during World War II but the first European to penetrate the territory was a gold prospector, Ted Eubank, leading whites away from the invading Japanese. Later a Japanese plane crashed in the forests of the Fore and then a U.S. plane too, events that the Fore remembered precisely. When the Japanese were finally evicted, Papua and New Guinea returned to the judicial control of Australia. The first government patrols arrived in the North Fore region in 1947, but civil administration was not firmly established until the late 1950s. In 1953, a patrol officer, J. R. McArthur, emerged with a strange report: a mysterious disease was afflicting the Fore people called *kuru,* from their word meaning "trembling from fear and cold." Two years later, Dr. Vin Zigas, a young Lithuanian physician, set off on a series of medical patrols to investigate. From his Australian government hospital in Kainantu in the center of the Eastern Highlands, he trekked for days climbing farther and farther into the ranges of the so-called "uncontrolled country" (areas with native populations not yet under civil administration). As he approached a large Fore village, he could sense something was dreadfully wrong. When he got closer he was appalled.

Some people were shaking uncontrollably; others could hardly walk. Limbs splayed sideways, then gave way without warning; small children who could not stand held tightly to their mothers' hands; others jerked spastically as they strove to remain upright. Adults leaned on heavy poles, while others could not support themselves even sitting down. Those lying helplessly on the ground showed signs of starvation: ribs contoured the chests, eye muscles had lost all tone and though the victims could hear and understand questions, they could not reply, for they could no longer speak. Those unafflicted were in stark contrast: though not tall they were strong and stoutly built; there were no signs of malnutrition and all appeared healthy, alert, and active.

Vin Zigas thought he was seeing victims of Parkinson's disease, a neurologic condition which progresses over the years. Soon he learned that though kuru began innocently, sometimes with a prolonged headache and minor loss of coordination, it progressed so rapidly that in less than three months the victims could walk only with difficulty. Soon they could no longer walk even with a stick as crutch and finally were unable to stand unassisted. After four months, a victim was totally prone, incapable of movement. Now they required constant care by a family member – usually a spouse or female child – who fed and washed them, and aspirated their mucus, which otherwise caused choking. They became prey to several infections that ranged from ulcerated sores to pneumonia. Gradually each victim slowly degenerated; the shivering and tremors gave way to complete loss of muscular and neural coordination; speech became disturbed and finally disappeared, then the capacity to swallow; within a year of the first obvious symptoms, the patient was dead.

In 1956, Zigas again returned to the Fore. He collected blood serum from twenty-six victims and a brain from one female, and despatched the specimens to the Walter and Eliza Hall Institute of Medical Research in Melbourne, Australia, along with a formal report. He described kuru as "probably a new form of encephalitis," a fatal brain infection, and asked for help. Sir Macfarlane Burnet, director of the Hall Institute, noted his comments and indicated that an investigator would be sent. In March 1957, someone did turn up, but he hadn't been sent by the Hall Institute. They didn't even know he was going to the kuru region and he wasn't even Australian. He was an American pediatrician and his name was D. Carleton Gajdusek.

Though only thirty-three, Gajdusek already had a considerable reputation – for an omnivorous curiosity, manic enthusiasm, ferocious energy, a prodigious capacity for knowledge, facility in languages, and deep interest in pediatrics and anthropology, especially in primitive cultures. Studying physics and mathematics in college at seventeen, he escaped from wartime draft into the Manhattan Project by entering Harvard Medical School at nineteen and specialized in pediatrics and neurology, haunting the wards of Boston's Children's Hospital, for the diseases of young people captivated him. There, while still a student, he worked in biophysical research on problems of survival in wartime: with John Edsall in developing purification of blood products for military and civilian casualties; and with James Gamble, on the water and carbohydrate requirements for those on life rafts awaiting rescue. Research with three scientific giants followed: Michael Heidelberger, Linus Pauling, and Max Delbrück; then it was back to Harvard to study with John Enders, a pioneer of polio viruses. The anecdotes that have come down from these youthful days echo with exhaustion and delight, fury and admiration. Such was the explosive nature of the young man with the crew-cut hair, that his professors nicknamed him "Atom Bomb Gajdusek."

In 1952, as a young virologist, he was drafted by the U.S. Army into the Korean War to study an epidemic of hemorrhagic fever which had struck American troops in Korea. Then he joined Joe Smadel, head of the Department of Virus and Rickettsial Diseases at the Walter Reed Army Medical Center in Washington, D.C. This was a crucially lucky move, because probably no other person could have tolerated Gajdusek's irritating combination of brilliance and impossible behavior. Even more crucial was Smadel's willingness to gamble: he never worried about the possibility of failure. As intelligent and strong-willed as his new colleague, Smadel

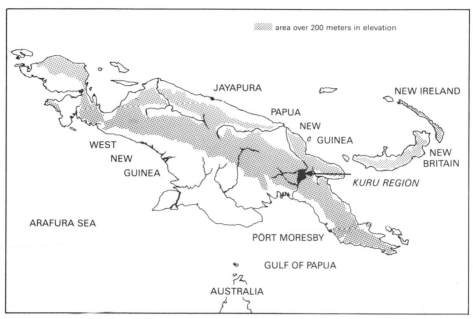

The kuru region (black shaded area) in Eastern Highlands Province of Papua New Guinea. (D. Carleton Gajdusek)

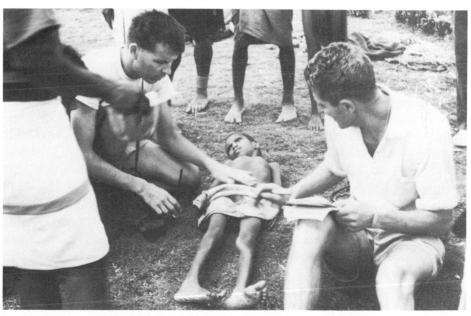

Dr. D. Carleton Gajdusek (left) and Dr. Vin Zigas (right) examine a South Fore child, victim of kuru, at Pintogori Kuru Hospital, Okapa Patrol Post. (D. Carleton Gajdusek; archive # 57-369B)

would spill his staff's blood all over the floor if need be, but fiercely protected them whether right or wrong.

There was no restraining Gajdusek. The imperatives of pediatrician-anthropologist, linguist-traveler, scientist-physician, always pressed. The itchy feet and restless intelligence took him to a variety of remote places, and this mobility puzzled his colleagues. Why not stay at home and climb to the top of the scientific ladder under the benevolent dictatorship of an established patron? But Gajdusek had one very specific and truly far-sighted reason for choosing his lonely path. The problem of humanity in isolation had always fascinated him. Small enclaves of people – lepers in restricted areas, gypsies in Transylvania, ascetics in Russia, Indians in South America and Mexico, nomadic peoples in central Asia, Stone Age tribes in New Guinea – he was eventually to visit them all – provide a unique opportunity for studying a whole variety of medical problems. Since such self-contained societies are not overlaid with extraneous shawls of "civilization," the scientific clues they yield are far more clear-cut than the clues to be discovered in larger, more diverse populations. Gajdusek believed that studying their epidemiology was bound to yield crucial scientific and medical dividends.

As soon as he could he resigned from Walter Reed and his army assignment, and disappeared to the Middle East in search of hemorrhagic fevers, plague, and rabies. Soon Joe Smadel was smothered with letters, a mélange of travel experiences, scientific questions, and medical information, a literary and scientific fallout that would drift over him for years to come. Gajdusek wrote as he spoke: everything poured out and vainly did Smadel instruct Gajdusek to "leave out the innumerable interesting conversational points about the travelogue aspects of the trip – and those about people, language, gossip, introspection, and indiscretions." He might as well have told Gajdusek to stop thinking.

By 1956, Gajdusek was in Melbourne, Australia, for a two-year period, as visiting investigator in viral genetics at the Walter and Eliza Hall Institute, working on the problem of immunity to hepatitis under the renowned virologist, later Nobel laureate, Sir Macfarlane Burnet. While there, he visited West New Guinea in 1956 and now, one year later, wanted to pass through the country again on his way back to Boston. Since he had planned a program devoted to child growth and development, and disease patterns in primitive cultures, to be centered at the Children's Medical Center at Harvard, he first wished to visit some primitive cultures. He would just move through Papua New Guinea once again with a patrol officer, Ian Burnet, the son of Sir Macfarlane Burnet, who was opening a new uncontrolled area in the highlands, and then would hasten home. Once in Port Moresby, however, he learned of the Fore's strange problem, and how medicine seemed to have a new, lethal, neurologic disease on its hands.

The challenge was irresistible: one night's talk with Vin Zigas was sufficient. Gajdusek abandoned his plans and, with Zigas, trekked south, from the subdistrict of Kainantu to the Okapa Patrol Post in the north of the Fore region, taking along some Fore who had been patients in Zigas's hospital and were returning home. Soon Gajdusek, too, was seeing, first-hand, the terrible ravages of kuru. His imagination was fired, his energies immediately engaged, and in March 1957 another big fat envelope landed on Joe Smadel's desk bearing the address: "Moke, at the Okapa Patrol Post; Fore, Kimi, Keiagana linguistic areas; Territory of Papua and New Guinea." The letter was an excited account of where Gajdusek was, what he was doing, and why. If Smadel had gambled on Gajdusek as a scientist when approached earlier for funds, for research in Iran, Afghanistan, and the Amazon jungles of Bolivia, Gajdusek, too, was now prepared to gamble and "stake his entire medical reputation" on investigating kuru.

In a second, exhilarated letter, on April 3, he insisted that "this is no wild goose chase, but a really big thing; everything in my medical training makes me confident." If necessary he could, and would, support the project with his own funds. But since he needed a few vital items urgently, could Smadel, please, find a temporary salary to pay for axes, beads, tobacco, and those other trading materials with which he could "purchase bodies (along with autopsy permission) and food for our patients." Then he could carry on long enough to "watch the evolution of a number of current cases to their fatal outcome."

He would stay for ten months and Smadel would receive volumes of letters requesting support of every kind: logistic, scientific, technical, financial, even diplomatic.

Diplomacy was called for because territorial imperatives were impinging. Gajdusek had written to Sir Macfarlane Burnet at the Walter and Eliza Hall Institute saying he would be at Okapa, and, if desired, he would send a kuru patient to Australia for a full clinical investigation. In a second letter he pointed out that Zigas's suggestion, encephalitis, was unlikely as an explanation for kuru because there were none of the characteristic symptoms of infections, such as fevers or sweats. He believed that epidemiologic and clinical investigations, starting with the known causes of neurologic diseases, would be the best tactic. The director of the

Public Health Service of the Territory of Papua and New Guinea, and Burnet at the Hall Institute, were left in no doubt that this American had started full-scale investigations in a frenzy of activity and they were incensed. Thus, on March 30, Gajdusek received an unwelcome radiogram. Since he had been given permission to visit the uncontrolled area of the highlands solely to go on patrol with Ian Burnet, and was not authorized to undertake work in the Fore area, he must leave. On ethical grounds he was requested to consider discontinuing his investigation into kuru. But Gajdusek had one great advantage, as he very well knew: possession is nine-tenths of the law anywhere, but nowhere more so than in the Eastern Highlands of New Guinea. He could be anywhere in an area of some thousands of square miles, totally out of reach.

He now began to study the progress of the disease in kuru patients from those Fore and Keiagana villages within one day's walk of the Okapa Patrol Post, the administrative center in the north of the area. But bacterial meningitis and many other acute medical problems were brought to him, and these had to be treated as well, with medicines sent in by Dr. Zigas from the Kainantu Hospital. Since there was no room in the rude aid post, Gajdusek took the really seriously ill children into the two-room hut in which he lived. Its dining table served a variety of functions — for study, clinical record-keeping, starting intravenous drips, doing lumbar punctures, surgery, as well as the sorting and studying of physiological specimens.

Soon there were more patients than could possibly be accommodated in his living quarters. With the enthusiastic support of Patrol Officer Jack Baker, who had been assigned to the kuru area, he organized the building of a small hospital. Constructed with native materials, the Pintogori Hospital featured an open hearth for warmth against the chilly nights at the 7,500 foot elevation. A simple laboratory was also made which Gajdusek and Zigas managed to stock with supplies and reagents. These came in by air to Kainantu, and Zigas sent them by cargo line from Kainantu to Pintogori. Later, Jack Baker, Vin Zigas, and Gajdusek arranged for the building of a permanent residence, to be used by Gajdusek and his many visitors. This place was a mere twenty-four foot square, with simple tables along the walls, but at least they could now eat without post-mortem specimens jostling their food.

The Fore were reluctant to stay in the hospital at first, but soon there were twenty-five patients — half children — and so Gajdusek now could regularly take samples of blood, urine, and feces as well as culture swabs of fungi, bacteria, and viruses. If patients agreed he would also

perform lumbar punctures to examine their cerebro-spinal fluid – a nerve-wracking procedure for both parties.

Therapeutically, he tried every procedure he could think of, and every promising medication he could obtain. Kuru patients received aspirin, vitamins, antibiotics, drugs against roundworms, and others against parasites, detoxifiers in case of metallic poisoning, drugs then on trial for multiple sclerosis, drugs which would calm convulsions. All were unsuccessful. If kuru was rare in adult men, perhaps their male hormones protected them, so he tried hormones like testosterone. Nothing worked. Some drugs he hoped to try, such as the tranquilizer, *Serpasil,* then used in the West for various types of neurologic tremors, were just not available. He finally had thirty-six kuru patients on a whole variety of therapeutic regimens; every one was useless. Such failures troubled him deeply, as he wrote to Smadel, "With the disease progressing relentlessly to speedy complete helplessness and death before our eyes, the Fore nation in turmoil because of it, and with ritual murders and savage killings in reprisals for kuru sorcery comprising the major administrative problems in the region at the moment, we certainly feel we should be doing more for our patients – even if these trials are based on the most remote chances of benefit. Therapeutically, we are licked. Sorcery seems as good an explanation for it (kuru) as any we can offer them."

Gajdusek now embarked on one of the most remarkable feats ever undertaken in medicine – a marathon trek around the Fore territory, mapping out the extent of kuru and drawing a complete clinical and epidemiologic profile of the disease, one that has never been superseded. During the next eight months, he walked nearly two thousand miles. Soon the Fore were gossiping about the white man who covered tremendous distances with his camp followers. When he ventured into other tribal areas, his "cargo line" entourage of small boys and young men went too. Most people patrolling in New Guinea took along men to carry the gear and to provide valuable links with the local people. A few adventurous boys too would come along for the sport. Children as young as five or ten would volunteer to carry Gajdusek's supplies and off each one would trot proudly bearing a camera or its tripod. Soon Gajdusek had amassed a team of boys who learned to communicate with him in Pidgin faster than he learned their native tongues. First they were translators of the eleven languages spoken by groups afflicted with kuru, then his field assistants, then hospital orderlies and, finally, medical assistants. The wives of two of the young men became the first nurses for the kuru patients. Other relatives lent a hand with all sorts of jobs. They constructed suspension bridges of rattan vines across the raging streams, or of tree trunks balanced precariously from one rocky outcrop to another. They built temporary sleeping shelters roofed with grass and the permanent house for Gajdusek at the Patrol Post. Without the support and kindness of these warm-hearted people Gajdusek would have been helpless. As it was, he achieved miracles.

His journeys began high in the mountains, dropped down to the edges of the rain forest where a deep, wide river separated the language groups, and back up again through grasslands and rain forests. Sometimes he went by himself, sometimes with Zigas, and sometimes with Patrol Officer Jack Baker – always trekking to the outlying villages, and returning to base with new patients, to evaluate the progress of long-term trials of new medications and the progression of their disease. His mobility is a crucial element in understanding the facts he spotted, the conclusions he reached, and the things he missed.

Why did Gajdusek choose to tackle the problem in this mobile way? An investigator in fiction needs minimal deductive powers to associate the bottle of prussic acid on the floor with the dead person lying beside it. In real life, however, diseases and deaths result from a complex interplay of many factors, so their causes rarely emerge clear-cut; neither do the clues to those causes. Since nothing whatever is obvious, many possibilities must be examined. Gajdusek and Vin Zigas faced a situation of monumental complexity – an unknown disease of epidemic proportions, with enigmatic symptoms, in an isolated and unfamiliar tribe. Scientists do have a well-tried method to cut through such jungles of complexity, and this Gajdusek was systematically applying. Essentially this meant garnering facts – whether environmental, clinical, pathological, or physiological. It meant collecting evidence, mapping the extent of the disease both within geographic space and within the social group, and sifting suggestions, ideas, and possibilities about the cause of kuru. He was to be constantly seeking correlations that would guide his quest, for patterns that would suggest a relation between the symptoms he could see and an underlying cause, as yet unseen.

There were several pressing questions to be answered at the outset. How far had kuru spread? Was it restricted to the Fore tribe or were their immediate neighbors afflicted? What were its geographic boundaries? How many people were affected? Was there any particular pattern to the disease within the tribe? By July, he knew there had been five hundred patients, with one hundred and fifty cases presently active, twenty-four of whom had died in the four months since he had arrived. But by August, when he and Zigas had tagged a further two hundred cases and fifty people were dead, he confirmed the pattern that was emerging. Kuru was rare in adult males: it predominated in adult females and in children of both sexes equally. It was restricted to an area of about one thousand square miles in range from three thousand to seven thousand feet above sea level. Though 50 percent of all deaths in any one year were due to the disease, only the Fore and those neighbors with whom they intermarried were afflicted. Most puzzling of all was the fact that not one of the many outsiders who had entered the Fore region since it opened up in the 1950s had ever contracted kuru.

As he moved around, generally remaining for one or two nights in each village, rumors began to spread and people now came to the foreign doctor. Supporting themselves with heavy sticks, some would trudge laboriously across country to intersect with his patrol while others would be carried. A poignant photograph shows a seven-year-old boy arriving at the kuru hospital at Pintogori lying on a rough stretcher of branches. The boy had been carried for two days across the mountains by youngsters of his own age. Patients with milder complaints also turned up, some requiring minor surgery. Trying to win the confidence of the people, Gajdusek treated everyone.

As he investigated and questioned and treated, Gajdusek was also ferreting for clues to the agent responsible, and he steadfastly believed that these *must* ultimately emerge from the epidemiologic data. Since the disease was occurring in clusters of people, the natural explanation was still an infection, most likely an acute viral one. But the classic symptoms never showed – no obvious fevers, sweats, or changes in white blood cells – nor any of the tell-tale signs of brain infection. All clinical tests – whether tested at Okapa by Gajdusek, or in Port Moresby, Australia, or the National Institutes of Health in the United States – gave no indications that bacterial, parasitic, fungal, or viral agents were at work. Most convincingly, samples from the bodies of kuru victims, whether ground up and injected into laboratory animals, or set up as tissue cultures at the Hall Institute by Gajdusek's former laboratory technician, Lois Larken, provoked nothing at all.

Factors in the environment were the next possibility. Many agents could be responsible, and many were considered – metallic poisons for a start – since some were known to promote brain diseases similar to kuru. The smoke from the Fore's fires, the ash from burned wood, the hot stones they cooked with, the thatch they built with, the animals they hunted, even the soil they stepped in, might contain poisonous metals. Off went these samples for analysis and testing. Blood, urine, feces, hair, and

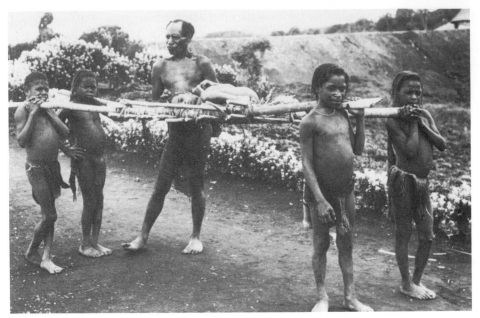

Yakurimba, aged 7, kuru victim from Agakamatasa village, South Fore, arriving at Pinto-gori Kuru Hospital on stretcher carried by his friends, after a two-day journey across the ranges separating village from Okapa Patrol Post.
(D. Carleton Gajdusek; archive # 57-195)

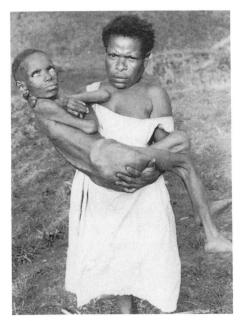

South Fore mother holds her kuru-afflicted daughter, in late stages of disease. The child is emaciated, having lost the ability to swallow.
(D. Carleton Gajdusek; archive # 57-XV-18)

fingernails, and autopsy tissues from kuru patients were also subjected to similar trace metal analysis. Perhaps the problem stemmed from something the Fore ate. A plant, manioc, that contains prussic acid was a likely candidate because it had been introduced into the Eastern Highlands at the same time as kuru had been detected. In August 1957, Lucy Hamilton, an expert on native nutrition from the Public Health Department in New Guinea, joined Gajdusek. For many months she lived with the women of Moke village, staying in the traditional Women's House, investigating the differences in diet between what the men ate and what the women and children ate. Off for screening went the leaves from bushes, bark from trees, pig and human flesh, all packed up in ten-pound bales. An enormous collection of those wild and cultivated plants, used by the Fore for food, medicine, and body paint, was sent to botanists in Lae, Adelaide, the U.S.A., and Europe for identification and determination of their alkaloid content. Once more the findings were totally negative: there were no toxic substances in the food. Next the drinking water was analyzed for harmful trace elements: there weren't any.

Kuru was clearly neither a disease of old age nor a natural consequence of senility, because mostly young adults and children were affected, but could it be simply mass hysteria? Gajdusek gave short shrift to such a view because genuine neurologic signs cannot be mimicked by hysteria. A few cases of hysteric mimicry of the disease were seen, but the people recovered suddenly and never showed true neurologic symptoms. Then, the director of psychiatry of Melbourne Hospital visited and pronounced definitively: Kuru was neither a psychotic nor a hysterical disease.

Cannibalism was the next candidate, the practice not being unusual in New Guinea. It would be a reason easily acceptable, for if kuru were an infection, cannibalism would provide a natural avenue for the passage of the agent from one person to another. When Gajdusek learned that the Fore people ate all tissues of only their close kinsmen, as an expression of sorrow, respect, and love for their dead, he recognized that this practice could easily transmit infections. But since the laboratory studies revealed no such infection, he fleetingly wondered whether eating someone else's brain might induce a build-up of self-sensitization in the eater's brain, similar to that which repeated injections of penicillin can induce? "It is a wild idea," he wrote, "but evidently this disease is a wild one." He had Lois Larkin look in kuru specimens for the crucial antibodies. There were none.

Only one possible causal candidate was left: heredity. As an explanation genetics was both reasonable and likely, for not only did outsiders never catch kuru, but the disease did run in families. Over the months of his marathon treks, as Gajdusek collected Fore genealogies, the genetic cause of kuru gradually came to dominate. Still, his diaries of that time reveal that, like a juggler, he kept all the possibilities in the air and was right to do so. He swung, week by week, from infection (which was quickly ruled out when the first pathology reports arrived), to the environment, to cannibalism, to genetics and, finally, back to infection again, still believing that a genetic predisposition might be behind the whole mystery. While both keeping all his options open and hedging all his bets, he was still a good scientist, for he remained agnostic; the evidence would not yet permit him to favor one hypothesis over the others.

In time, Gajdusek came to believe that the problem had defeated him, and soon his morale was at low ebb. After struggling for months he was facing the possibility that he had taken a colossal gamble and lost. He had neither discovered the cause of kuru nor done anything for the patients – and they knew it. Now the Fore were beginning to be skeptical, impatient, and even antagonistic. All he had to show for his marathon efforts was a plethora of notebooks and clinical records about a strange new disease. So on August 6, 1957, he wrote to Joe Smadel, "kuru has us licked."

During August, Gajdusek's spirits plummeted, but still he kept going, even though his practical difficulties had worsened. He battled furiously, under most primitive conditions, to keep sterile the clinical specimens for microbial and biochemical studies; to get samples to the United States quickly and reports on them back without delay; to keep open his lines of communication; to dampen down the territorial conflicts that continued to erupt, as the outraged Australians learned that kuru specimens were going to the United States. His impotence in the face of a disease whose mysteries he could not fathom and whose victims he could not help, weighed heavily. The exhausting physical and psychological conditions under which he labored, now verging on the dangerous, threatened to overwhelm him, for he was flooded with compassion for the desperate plight of the people he had come to love and in whose company he felt truly happy.

There was, he saw, only one positive outcome so far: a series of kuru brains were now safely in Australia and in the United States. He had been lucky to obtain them and this always had been his main preoccupation. But it had taken so long to get the first brain that, from the start, he was thoroughly pessimistic about obtaining any at all. The deaths that actually occurred in his very first weeks in the highlands had not been discovered for a long time ~~(illegible handwritten note overlay)~~ ad been in the territory for two months, he ~~had six...~~ it not one had died and though there were ~~six te...~~ al, it was impossible to remain there waitin~~g, just to be present at the mo~~ment of death, for this would disrupt othe~~r vital studies. There were othe~~r reasons for his pessimism. "It is," he wr~~ote, "almost impossible to con~~vince the natives to stay with us as death ap~~proaches, for they want abov~~ all else to be on home ground at death. Th~~us, they are willing to let us tr~~y every possible procedure and therapeuti~~c test until they think the pati~~ents are near terminal. Then they must be ~~at home – often days of rugged~~ trails away. However we are hanging on t~~o a few near-terminal cases, an~~d hoping to be able to secure autopsies wi~~thout disrupting the confiden~~ce we have laboriously won from the peopl~~e." Thus when, in mid-May, h~~e did that first autopsy on the small boy against the counterpoint of a tropical storm, he despatched the brain to Australia along with this warning. The specimen should be treated as if it were the only one they would ever receive.

His caution was wise. Though other deaths did occur up to the end of May, he was unable to obtain any more brains and was acutely aware that the Fore were not people he should push.

They are proud, and have their own ideas, which are most intelligent; and although they have conceded that I can cure their meningitis and pneumonia, they have decided that this magic (kuru) is too strong for me and that my prolonging life by treating and controlling decubitus ulcers is no blessing at all. They want to die at home; and once fully incapacitated, they want to die as quickly as possible. With such apparent hopeless neurological disease, you cannot blame them. Since we have done lumbar punctures on over fifty (repeatedly on some) and loaded them with painful shots (everything from crude liver extract and cortisone to parenteral antibiotics) without effect – and they know it – I have only more respect for their "hands off" attitude. But, to humor me and repay my many miles of mountain-climbing to track them down, they haul litters over miles of cliff-faced and precipitous jungle slopes to bring the patients in for another shot at our therapeutic trials and experimental poking. I admire and respect them thoroughly.

At the end of May another opportunity arose and Gajdusek seized it. A middle-aged woman died in his hospital from a classic case of kuru. Following explicit instructions sent from NIH, he and his assistant did not slice the brain but dropped it whole into 50 percent formol saline solution. Carried first by the bush pilots who connected with Qantas Airways, the brain traveled on the biweekly KLM Airlines service to Holland, and reached the United States via Europe having gone around the world. But Gajdusek continued to worry: kuru brains were not a commodity upon the open market, he wrote, nor would they ever be. His colleagues at NIH were lucky to get them and so precious were they that he needed assurance from Smadel that the brains would reach only those scientists prepared to study them properly.

More autopsies followed, all done under the most appalling conditions: Gajdusek had neither tools nor refrigeration nor some of the chemicals he wanted for fixing the specimens. He operated surrounded by people whose reactions he could not gauge, no matter that he had previously established a warm relationship and now spoke their language. Talking, questioning, examining, and treating them was one thing. Asking them to submit to the pricks of needles for blood and the stab of tubes for spinal fluid, was another. For them to watch the crude opening of a skull and the extraction and preservation of a brain in strong-smelling formaldehyde in the white hours of that first stormy morning had been a most awesome sight which rattled the Fore's confidence. So every time another autopsy was performed, their suspicions were once more aroused. Some widows suspected that he took the brains so others might eat them, and though quite tranquil about most aspects of post-mortems, they did not like the opening of the head. Only by carefully sewing back the retracted scalp to restore the appearance of the corpse to "normal" were they comforted. Yet the really upsetting factor was to die away from their home villages. However, Gajdusek knew he had to press the people to obtain more brains and yet still more. Though he still had no clues to the cause he continued to believe that kuru was one of the most important problems in medical research. "It has," he wrote to Smadel, "all the earmarks of one that may give a real lead into chronic degenerative neurologic diseases."

In June, he performed more autopsies and got one brain from a small girl and another from a middle-aged woman. Gajdusek was out on patrol when the girl had died, but his Fore medical assistant followed his instructions meticulously: the autopsy was done properly and the brain dropped into the formaldehyde fixative that Gajdusek had prepared earlier. Two more deaths occurred in the second week in July, and the brains were out of the skulls within the hour. Still more brains were obtained in August, and Gajdusek's convictions as to the medical importance of kuru intensified. "That this is the best site in the world for study of chronic progressive degenerative disease of the CNS [central nervous system] at the moment, I am fully convinced. . . ." he wrote, "If we can't 'crack' kuru — with hundreds of cases available for full study in any three- to six-month period — I see little hope for Parkinsonism, Huntington's Chorea, multiple sclerosis, etc."

During August Gajdusek's relationship with the Fore subtly shifted, and some of the families became angry. Soon the moment arrived when either no more brains were available, or the conditions under which they could be obtained were greatly changed. In order to continue to obtain specimens, Gajdusek invoked his powers of persuasion. Between August 25 and September 22 he managed to keep four terminal patients around his base and, when they had died, perform autopsies on them obtaining the brains from some of them. "It is most difficult," he admitted, and one month later wrote

... it looks as though further autopsy materials may be unobtainable. The natives have given up on our medicine; they know damn well it does not work, and I am fighting [verbal battles in Fore], bribing, cajoling, begging, pleading, and bargaining for every opportunity to see a patient, and strenuously working tongue muscles for hours, for every day we get a patient to stay in the hospital, accept therapeutic trials, etc., etc. Vin is sick and tired of the "duress of personality" which is required to pressure every case into our care, and I do not like the effort. I am willing to keep up the push, using every ruse short of actual duress by force and authority – *that* we cannot contemplate.

But now the barriers seemed insurmountable, his ignorance total and his impotence absolute. It was clearly time to move to the laboratory for further study of collected specimens, so by December 8 Gajdusek was winding things down. His detailed epidemiological data filled many notebooks and nearly one thousand cards; he had complete clinical observations on over two hundred kuru patients, a hundred of whom had died, and he was eagerly awaiting the neuropathological reports on the brains already despatched. As the last days of 1957 ran their course, he shipped his case records and field studies, his correspondence files, and all the other records on which future work would be based. On December 30 he did two final post-mortems, using the very crudest of instruments, since all the others had been sent down to Kainantu for Vin Zigas.

Sadly, reluctantly, and baffled as ever, Gajdusek prepared to depart. What leads, he pleaded in a letter to Joe Smadel, could the scientists at Bethesda give him about a causal agent for this mysterious disease that, on first exposure, generated absolutely no symptoms at all, whose incubation clearly preceded the illness by months or, probably, many years? He may have been facing failure of his self-imposed mission, but Gajdusek was just at the start of a long love affair with the mystery of kuru and its victims. He remained obsessed with the problems, and this obsession and his deep compassion for the Fore, never waned. Over the years he would adopt three dozen Melanesian and Micronesian children, educate them in America, and start them off in a variety of careers. It was during the time of his great ten-month "walkabout" that the binding occurred, when lines of affection were laid down and relationships cemented. Gajdusek joined that eminent roll of scientists – Miklukho MacLay, Bronislaw Malinowski, Beatrice Blackwood, Camilla Wedgewood, Margaret Mead, Mervin Megitt, Andrew and Marilyn Strathern – who developed enduring bonds of affection with the people of Papua New Guinea.

As departure drew near, Gajdusek worked obsessedly: devising a system to monitor kuru over the long term; writing reports and letters to Australia and Washington; grabbing additional specimens whenever he could – food samples, blood, urine, fingernails, hair, brains, tissues, "a good long piece of spinal cord"; planning the studies to be continued in his absence; shipping reels of film in cans and autopsy specimens in jars; coping with the future politics of who would be responsible for kuru and with the present ones over proper procedures. The Public Health Department of New Guinea was pained to learn that Gajdusek would be taking his field records, but he rightly insisted that not only did they belong to him but it would be impossible for anyone else either to decipher his writing or to organize his notes. In any case, carbon copies of everything had been made, which had already been thoroughly mined by university students, as materials for their dissertations.

Such snarling scraps simmered for some time to come, and Gajdusek constantly has had to live with the accusation that he "stole" the disease. The truth is that – in contrast to the more sedate methods of other scientists – his brilliant assessment of kuru's medical significance combined with his extremely swift scientific reflexes, his insistence on immediate action, and his unremitting energy, enabled him to come in first and to stay there. Yet, as he packed, it seemed that a comprehensive medical record would be the only lasting achievement of the exhausting ten-month experience.

Smadel kept urging him to hurry back, but still Gajdusek delayed until mid-January 1958, so as to brief the Australian scientists now coming into New Guinea to study kuru. He finally returned to Bethesda, having stopped over in West New Guinea, Malaya, India, the Soviet Union, Finland, and Sweden. Smadel had kept his promises and a special job, in the Office of the Director of the National Institute of Neurological Diseases and Blindness of the NIH, was waiting. So, in a very "sheltered" role as head of a small laboratory in Collaborative and Field Research Gajdusek moved his planned study of "Child Growth and Development and Disease

Patterns in Primitive Cultures" to the NIH in Bethesda, Maryland. By August 1958, he was once more back in New Guinea among the people he loved. The cause of kuru was as elusive as ever.

Yet though Gajdusek could not appreciate how formidable his achievement really was, the first chapter in unraveling the mystery of kuru was complete. As Shirley Lindenbaum, the anthropologist who years later would make a significant contribution to the problem, said,

This was an extraordinary epidemiological survey, of a kind that only a person like Gajdusek could pull off, because of his mad energy and his mad adventurousness . . . [his willingness] to disregard the necessity to get permission from the authorities to do certain things, as well as to go in and out of the areas. . . . he was going to be a headache for them in any case. He doesn't get permission for any of these journeys, of course, nor for any of the medical procedures – he just goes off and does them.

Not until eight years later was the full potential of Gajdusek's extraordinary achievement realized and his predictions about kuru magnificently fulfilled. The clues to success *did* indeed lie in the recesses of the brains he had despatched to the U.S., and kuru's significance to other neurologic disorders was *vital*. Four separate elements would be provided by other scientists and added to Gajdusek's first clinical and epidemiologic studies. Taken together, these elements – an astute connection, perceived by a pathologist, a perceptive suggestion made by a veterinarian, some brilliant observations by two anthropologists, along with unique and pioneering experiments by Gajdusek's laboratory team – would finally enable scientists to comprehend the mystery of kuru.

The pathologist's report on the first brain had arrived in New Guinea in June 1957 and was singularly unhelpful. Perhaps there were slightly fewer types of one particular cell in the cerebellum, but that was all. A month later a preliminary note on the second brain also arrived, and its observations were perhaps more encouraging but no more illuminating. Though no traces of inflammation nor infection had been found, and though bacterial and viral theories had to be discarded once again, the pathologist did report significant neural degeneration in several areas. Gajdusek had to wait another two months, until September 1957, before a full report arrived, which, though it still shed no light on the cause of kuru, did make an intriguing link, one that was eventually to prove crucial.

When Gajdusek had finally left the Eastern Highlands in the winter of 1958, several brains were already at NIH. One gloomy March day, Dr. Igor Klatzo, a neuropathologist, came into his office and found sixteen jars of human brains lined up on the bench. Alongside was an untidy bundle of papers – the garbled messages and scrawled field notes of one Carleton Gajdusek whom he had never met – and written instructions to report on the pathology of the specimens. Klatzo was annoyed. He had moved to NIH solely to do experiments, not pathology, so he went to his scientific director, Dr. Milton Schein, and protested. Was it really necessary to examine these messy specimens? Instructions had come from on high, he was told succinctly. Both Joe Smadel and the director of the NIH had insisted the brains be quickly investigated.

Reluctantly Klatzo started work. Grossly the specimens showed no special abnormalities and four were in such a poor state that they were useless for microscopic examination. Twelve were in remarkably good condition considering how they had been obtained and that they had traveled round the globe wrapped in muslin soaked in formalin. Klatzo and his technician began their routines, preparing each brain in exactly the same way: photographed first, then impregnated with wax, then sliced by a microtome into microscopically thin sections which were placed on slides and stained with gold chloride. This was the standard procedure for pathological investigation of brain tissue. When, at last, Klatzo examined the sections under the microscope, he saw nothing unusual at all, only some minor degeneration of nerve cells. He felt insecure about this negative finding, for if Joe Smadel had been so insistent presumably something odd should be present. But he couldn't see anything unusual.

Klatzo's interest flickered, however, when he began detailed microscopic examination. Interest changed to high excitement as he suddenly realized that he was looking at something never before described in Western medicine: "a strong and diffuse proliferation of astrocytic brain cells." He had some new Nichol prisms that directed polarized light through his microscope and, just fiddling, casually flipped the switch that directed his light through the eyepiece. Now he saw something he had never seen in a human brain before – quantities of solid plaques, of beautiful colors, making tracks through the brain tissue like strange footprints in new snow. This was highly puzzling, so Klatzo began a systematic investigation and in the weeks that followed became more intrigued. Clearly something was badly awry, for not only were there unusual plaques but also spider webs of multiplying brain cells, astrocytes. These are not uncommon, but in the kuru brains there were far too many of them. Finally, there were gaping white holes where nerve cells should have been. He could make no sense of the picture at all.

Once his investigation was finished, he had to write a report, and then a proper scientific paper. He was baffled. The usual paragraphs describing what he had, what he had done with what he had, how he had proceeded, what he had looked for, and what he thought he saw, were easy enough. But there is always a section headed "Discussion" and, he recalls, "I was really sweating on that. I couldn't think of what to say. I tried first to eliminate every etiological agent whose morphology I knew in the brain. Whatever the problem was, it didn't look to me as though it was caused by toxicity, or by heredity, or by infection. So I was forced to think very hard about what the condition did resemble, and suddenly, something clicked." He remembered an observation made many years before in another fatal degenerative neurologic disease, a rare condition with only twenty cases reported in the medical literature. Burrowing through textbooks kept from his student days in Germany, he found the references. Then he did an extensive search through the German literature, at that time the most comprehensive on neurologic degenerative diseases. Soon he had the monograph that described the disease he had remembered: Creutzfeldt-Jakob disease (CJD). This condition too, provoked similar brain changes — astrocytic proliferation, gaping holes, and strange plaques. And that is what he mentioned in his discussion. But since no one knew what caused CJD either, this comment still shed no light on kuru, so the Fore continued to die. The connection Klatzo had made was brilliant nonetheless, and provided the first decisive elements in unraveling the mystery.

By now interest about kuru in the public press was intense. During 1957, journalists and cameramen had descended en masse upon the Eastern Highlands, writing accounts that, Gajdusek believed, were distorted and garbled and that provoked in him a long-lasting antipathy to the media. But in the spring of 1959, the Wellcome Institute in London, a medical foundation concerned with the history of medicine, mounted an exhibition on kuru at the Burroughs Wellcome Museum, based on material he had sent over. It contained photographs of the terrain, patients, and the microscopic pathology of kuru, done by Klatzo. By chance, a young American veterinarian dropped in. Bill Hadlow had been seconded to the British Ministry of Agriculture and was working at Compton, Berkshire, as a pathologist in a large program on animal research. He had arrived during a critical period of focused effort, as scientists tried to reproduce experimentally in goats an infectious disease, scrapie, whose ravages were causing great financial losses in sheep.

Hadlow specialized in this disease, which was, and still is, a terrible menace for sheep owners. It is so infectious that sick animals must be slaughtered at once or the disease spreads through the flock like wildfire. Animals genetically related to diseased sheep are also slaughtered, even though healthy, because the infection can be transmitted both from one to another generation and across a population. Hundreds of thousands of sheep still die from scrapie every year, but no one has ever discovered exactly how it spreads. The classic symptoms include uncontrollable trembling and, in some unfortunate beasts, the torture of continual itching.

British sheep farmers had been plagued for years and by the 1950s scrapie had spread to the United States, and the U.S. Department of Agriculture was compelled to take action. Since it was suspected that the source of infection was Suffolk breeding rams imported into the U.S.A. via Canada, the trade was embargoed. No one was happy about this edict: the sheep industry in the United States wanted the breed and Britain wanted the exports. The ban triggered renewed British investigations and scrapie research programs were set up at Compton as well as at the Mardon Veterinary Institution in Edinburgh. Having initiated the ban, the U.S. Department of Agriculture nevertheless wanted to be helpful, and that is why Bill Hadlow had been sent to England.

Dr. Hadlow had already spent years on the mysteries of scrapie. The disease was most unusual: whatever the causal agent, it could take up to four years to incubate. Although infected animals looked perfectly healthy until the first symptoms appeared, it was the central nervous system that was finally affected. Scientists suspected viruses because scrapie could be induced in laboratory animals by injecting them with cell-free filtrates of tissues from dead sheep. This revealed that the agent had properties that set it totally apart from all other known infectious agents: it could withstand high temperatures, even half an hour in boiling water, which inactivates most viruses; it was resistant to formaldehyde, which kills most bacteria; it could remain quiescent for months before producing symptoms. Agents that act stealthily and produce "slow" infections had surfaced before in veterinary medicine, but what really set them apart from usual infections, such as those that caused flu, was the ominous fact that the viruses never wholly disappeared. In familiar infections the whole process is self-limiting: once a full immune defense is mounted, the virus is rapidly obliterated. But with slow infections the agent was masked, latent, in a silent carrier state; when awakened it was slow to act, progressively destructive, never completely eradicated by the immune system, and always fatal.

In the spring of 1959, an American colleague passing through Britain made a suggestion that had dramatic consequences. Hadlow might find it worthwhile to visit the exhibition at the Burroughs Wellcome Museum. Slowly Hadlow moved through the hall, past the photographs of the patients and the printed details of the Fore people, past explanations

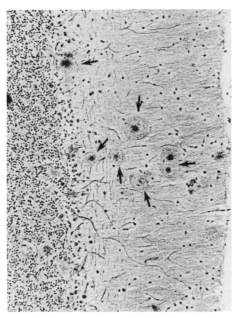 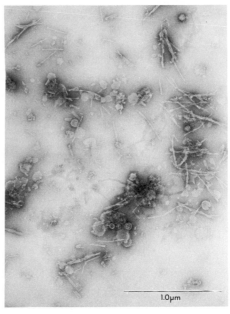

Light micrograph of the cerebellum from a case of Gerstmann-Straussler syndrome, a disease that shares some features with Creutzfeldt-Jakob disease and Alzheimer's disease. Characteristically, there are many plaques (arrows).
(Institute for Basic Research in Developmental Disabilities, Staten Island, NY # 2–6)

Electron micrograph of scapie-associated fibers isolated from the brain of a scrapie-infected mouse.
(Institute for Basic Research in Developmental Disabilities, Staten Island, NY # 5138)

of the symptoms and details of the investigations on tissues shipped back for study. Finally, he read Klatzo's pathology report and saw his microphotographs of the kuru brain sections. As he absorbed the information, Hadlow was overtaken by a sense of *déja vu*, for he was seeing changes he had been observing for years. The similarity between the symptoms in both kuru and scrapie was extraordinary. The brain changes were strikingly the same, for the photographs of the kuru lesions showed the same patterns as in scrapie: degeneration of nerve cells and great white spaces in the brain. Ever since scrapie was first described in 1899 it has been the presence of these great spaces, the vacuoles, that has been the pathological hallmark.

The progress of the two diseases was similar too. Both the Fore and the sheep showed identical first symptoms: excitability and tremors of the head. As the disease progressed, both became unsteady, the limbs splayed out and they could not stand. The same profound behavioral changes also occurred: humans and sheep seemed to be lost; they could no longer recognize familiar features and were completely out of touch with their surroundings. Scrapie was considered a dementia of sheep; kuru was clearly a slowly progressive dementia of the Fore, and during a period of three to six months, both diseases followed their relentless, fatal, downhill course.

There was, however, one puzzling dissimilarity between kuru and scrapie. Scrapie was known to be an infectious disease: its infectious nature had been experimentally proved by the French scientists Cuille and Chelle in 1933. Yet no one believed kuru *was* infectious.

As Hadlow strolled back and forth, looking at the exhibits and digesting the facts about kuru, the similarities between the two diseases seemed so obvious that he found it hard to believe that kuru, too, was not a subacute, slow but ultimately fatal *infection* of the central nervous system. The exhibition listed references to the few published papers and Hadlow proceeded to the library to study them. The more he read, the more convinced he became that the parallels between the two diseases were crucially significant. He was thus prepared to make a connection that seemed not only utterly natural but the only possible one.

One other fact encouraged him to make this connection publicly, one that would take many people by surprise, Gajdusek included. Even though it was now more than two years since Gajdusek had returned from New Guinea, arguments about the cause of kuru were still raging and all the old theories were still being tossed around. But Hadlow realized that insofar as Gajdusek's team suspected kuru was an infection, they had all used the wrong model. Experimentally they were approaching kuru as they would any acute, viral infection: they were inoculating their animals correctly, but waiting only a few weeks – at the most a month – for the effect. Because the infection was slow, however, nothing *could* happen within that time. Since nothing happened, the scientists concluded that kuru could not be an infection, but Hadlow knew that this did not follow.

He believed that they should apply to kuru the proven successful experimental techniques of scrapie research. For experimental subjects one could not, of course, use humans, but what animal *could* one inoculate with the tissue of kuru victims and, if one was prepared to wait – perhaps even years – expect to see an infection develop? The only possible candidate he felt was a nonhuman laboratory primate.

Dr. Hadlow wrote to Gajdusek along these lines on July 6, 1959. Gajdusek, then in New Guinea, received the forwarded letter and replied, asking for more information on scrapie. He was instantly alerted to the possibility of long incubation periods, already known in bacterial, fungal, and parasitic infections, and now in viral infections too. Then Hadlow, having corresponded with Gajdusek about the details of kuru, in his turn wrote a Letter to the Editor, published in the British medical journal, *The Lancet,* on September 5, 1959.

Once again, this connection – the second of the four crucial elements in the solution of the mystery – was brilliant. But in being able to make this, Hadlow had two advantages over all other investigators. First, he approached the problem with a mind neither clouded by previous thinking nor exhausted by repeated and futile excursions into etiological cul-de-sacs. Second, he was totally familiar with a disease of identical pattern.

On November 23, 1959, Hadlow was in the U. S. on a nationwide lecture tour, talking to sheep farmers about controlling scrapie. He had cabled Gajdusek that he was coming and hoped to meet with him. But by the time he left England he had had no response. His first lecture was in Washington, D.C., and he saw a man at the back of the hall, who stood throughout, who made no comments, but who, at the end, came up, introduced himself and commented on the *Lancet* letter. It was Carleton Gajdusek.

From then on, Hadlow corresponded sporadically with Gajdusek and in the spring of 1961 Gajdusek wrote, saying that they were putting together a research program. This would involve inoculation of chimpanzees and other primates with kuru tissue. The animals would then be held for long-term observation. He hoped Hadlow would consider joining them at the NIH. But by then Hadlow was permanently ensconced in the Rocky

Mountain Laboratory at the University of Montana and setting up his own research program on scrapie. Loving the problem and Montana almost equally, he declined and Gajdusek continued to search for someone to run his new primate section.

In June of that year, Gajdusek made a trip to Sigurdson's laboratory in Keldur, Iceland, the source of the concept of slow virus infections in veterinary medicine. There Paul Paulsson showed him their work, the Icelandic form of scrapie, *reda,* and other slow infections of sheep. He also visited the Mardon Institute of Edinburgh, Scotland, and the Compton laboratories in England and immediately resolved to use a "Noah's Ark" approach to the problem. He would inoculate with kuru brain tissue many species of laboratory animals, including monkeys and chimpanzees and observe them for at least five years. Following the same path of reason he suspected that many other non-inflammatory brain degenerative diseases might also be slow virus infections. He would simultaneously inoculate other animals with brain tissues of patients who had died from multiple sclerosis, or amyotrophic lateral sclerosis, or Alzheimer's disease, or Parkinson's disease.

Once back at NIH, he planned these inoculation projects in collaboration with Dr. Tony Morris. In order to house and care for the large laboratory primates, they sought better animal quarters than the cramped virus laboratory in the basement of Building 8 on the NIH campus. Through Dr. Carlton Hermann, the virologist of the Fish and Wildlife Preserve at Patuxent, Maryland, they were given permission to keep their animals out there. But Tony Morris was leaving so another virologist was sought to supervise the Patuxent laboratory.

Dr. Clarence Joseph Gibbs, Jr. – a small, round, cheerful Southern bachelor – came into kuru with as little enthusiasm as Igor Klatzo. He first ran into Carleton Gajdusek in 1951 when they were both working at the Walter Reed Army Medical Center, but while Gajdusek disappeared to exotic places, Gibbs simply moved to another part of the building. Eight years later while working on tropical neurology at NIH, he told his boss, Joe Smadel, that he was leaving for Brazil. Smadel said, "Goddamn it, you are not going to Brazil." So Gibbs asked, "Where am I going, then?" "You're going to Gajdusek," came the reply. "You are going to give stability to an otherwise unstable program."

Gibbs, most reluctant to leave the safe waters of conventional virology for a voyage on the stormy seas of kuru navigated by the flamboyant Gajdusek, argued for a whole day. When finally Gibbs succumbed,

Smadel said, "Either you're going to have a golden negative in this program or a golden positive – and I suspect a golden positive."

So began Joe Gibbs's collaboration with Carleton Gajdusek, one that has lasted twenty-five years and which works magnificently, he says, because not only are they total opposites but they have never shared the same laboratory. "I am on the fourth floor and he on the fifth; I stay at home and he travels. I was dealing with Smadel who was a genius and with Gajdusek who is also a genius, but I managed to survive by staying far enough away from both so that I could do my own work quietly. The first thing I had to do was build up the laboratory at the Patuxent Research Center."

Five thousand acres of secluded park in the Maryland countryside comprise the Patuxent Wildlife Center. Twenty-five miles from Bethesda, it is beautiful, rolling countryside of woods, streams and lakes and many, many mosquitoes. The laboratory built here was, Gibbs believes, the most important location in the whole kuru story. His task was simple: to transmit kuru to experimental animals. Its execution would be formidable however, and this was one reason for his reluctance to leave conventional viruses for unconventional ones. No doubt, kuru presented a wonderfully exciting challenge – a new disease in an isolated Stone Age tribe, of epidemic proportions that was spreading fast. But it showed none of the characteristics of an infection; yet Gibbs's mission was precisely to demonstrate that it was an infection. Not only would his scientists have to stretch their imaginations to the utmost, but they would be living with the knowledge that every single previous attempt had been a complete failure. And, as Joe Gibbs said, faced with the reality of a lot of negative experiments, where do you go? Still, the challenge was one virtually impossible to decline. For "implicit in it was the belief that if you're bright enough, smart enough, dedicated enough, you'll eventually find the answer."

Two caretakers for the animals were recruited. Gibbs soon expanded his research quarters from the single laboratory their program had been allocated into the next one, then on he went, up the corridor, acquiring more space until eventually he had a sizable scientific empire.

Persuading Joe Smadel to support the program had not been easy, for keeping a colony of chimpanzees and other primates for years and years would not be cheap, and, moreover, the complicated research program they proposed to him was based on the suggestion of a veterinarian of whom no one had ever heard. But once he was convinced, Smadel's influence proved decisive yet again: money and space were quickly found. All was chaos at first. Hadlow recalls dropping into the laboratory one day in August of 1961 to see only three infant chimpanzees grinning at him. But new, outdoor housing was soon built at Patuxent, with cages set in serial order and indoor and outdoor runs. The scientists worried a great deal about boredom among their animals, for a chimpanzee in a cage with nothing to do will start unraveling the wire, or take the oak benches, several inches thick, and reduce them to splinters. Fifty-four animals would finally be housed and being the caretaker was no sinecure. On one occasion the chimps unlocked all the cage doors. They didn't leave, the winter day being bitter, but the squirrel monkeys did, and they had to be rounded up. One resolutely stayed in the trees and had to be shot. Problems there may have been, but Joe Gibbs nostalgically recalls those days as the happiest and most productive ever.

Gajdusek and Gibbs were poised to try something never before attempted in science: to put human material into nonhuman primates and to wait for five years. Then either transmission of the disease would have taken place or they would have yet one more negative result and wonder where to go. In 1962, they ground up brains of kuru victims and injected these into a rhesus monkey and in 1963, into chimpanzees imported from Sierra Leone. Then they began the long wait. Thus was initiated the third crucial element in solving the kuru mystery.

It was now five years since Carleton Gajdusek had arrived in the Eastern Highlands, but the Fore tribe had not been ignored during this time: Gajdusek had visited them each year. In 1961, when the laboratory experiments were being planned, two young anthropologists went to the Fore to study kuru from a fresh standpoint. The American, Robert Glasse, had already worked in New Guinea but his Australian wife, Shirley Lindenbaum, had never been into the field. They were sent by Dr. John Bennett of the Department of Genetics at Adelaide University, a specialist in mathematical genetics who was convinced that kuru was caused by the presence of a single, dominant gene. Some medical students had already collected Fore pedigrees, but Bennett's critics were unimpressed by these efforts, insisting that anthropologists would garner such information far more effectively.

Before they left the two young people met all scientists in Australia interested in the genetic aspect of kuru research. Though they would be given a free hand, it was nevertheless made clear that they were to concentrate on genetics and harvest as much genealogical information as possible. They flew from Australia to Port Moresby, then in a small aircraft on to Kainantu in the Eastern Highlands. Here a government Land Rover was waiting to load their nine months' supplies and drive them to the Okapa Station, headquarters of the subdistrict in which the Fore lived and kuru occurred. They stayed overnight with Dr. Andrew Gray, the resident physician, and next day drove the eighteen miles to Purosa. Halfway down they stopped at a most appealing place, a valley where there was a high incidence of kuru. Robert Glasse spoke to the local Fore youths who had learned the lingua franca, Pidgin, who were urging them to live in the village of Wanitabe. But first, they continued on, to discuss matters with the resident European missionary at Purosa before returning to discuss the matter with the Fore once more.

The next day they moved into a tiny hut in the village, and on day 3, with Glasse as the designer and the Fore the builders, began their house – just one large room, a separate outside *haus kuk* place, and an outside latrine. During the six weeks of building, Shirley Lindenbaum started to master Pidgin and the ritual greetings, but most important, she was establishing contacts with the women by being with them while they worked, at home, or in their gardens. Like house-building this activity was aimed at forging those warm relationships upon which the success of their work would depend. Robert Glasse was taking the lead at this point because it was all so new to his wife. She was having to adapt to so many things: she couldn't speak the language; she feared that the people's gestures were aggressive; she had to become accustomed to the women fondling her all over to satisfy their curiosity about how she was made; she had never used a latrine before; she didn't like spiders; she was terrified of snakes. But soon she had learned to walk carefully, particularly on patrols, and especially in one region notorious for its small, lethal, death adders. The Fore recognized the dangers and always made Robert Glasse march third, for he was wearing boots. "The first person wakens the snake," they said. "On arrival of the second he coils; with the third he strikes." Lindenbaum was made to march sixth.

Some two hundred Fore lived in the village, friendly, hospitable, cheerful people, and soon the interviewing began – all very informally. People would visit the anthropologists' house at night, would be offered tea or soup, and the tape recorder would be turned on. Shirley Lindenbaum's skills as a stenographer were invaluable: every evening she reconstructed the interviews in a frenzy of writing. By the fourth month they were collecting data, finding out who was living in which houses, and mapping their kinships. Glasse also concentrated on questions of political organization; Shirley Lindenbaum gleaned a variety of information from the women about marriage patterns. From time to time, as occasion demanded – a marriage or death ceremony – they would go on patrol. They never pushed the Fore about kuru but just let the topic surface when it would. But they were garnering information about its impact on family structures – how these were now changing, who was caring for the orphans, what were the other social consequences of the disease. The people were not at all reluctant to talk, for this was a terrible time: the plague had reached dreadful proportions and morale was plummeting fast.

The Fore told them about many other things besides: about the foreign doctor who walked tremendous distances with an entourage of young boys, and about cannibalism. Although it was now totally forbidden under a government edict issued in the 1950s and also discouraged by the missionaries, and indeed had almost vanished, the Fore discussed cannibalism quite openly. There was little in their region, they said, but to the south, a few communities still surreptitiously disposed of the odd body in this way. Much to their surprise, the anthropologists learned that it was the women who were primarily involved. It was this fact that triggered the possibility of a connection between cannibalism and kuru.

More significantly at this stage, the two quickly realized that the genealogic information they had amassed was exploding the genetic hypothesis for kuru. Soon other, historical, data reinforced this conviction. The Fore were saying that kuru hadn't been around long: fifty years ago, there had been none. If true, this fact would be totally incompatible with any genetic hypothesis. Could they rely on what the Fore were remembering? Gajdusek and others said, "No," insisting that although primitive, illiterate people have memory of events in their own lifetime, their historical sense was not comparable to ours. So one should not reconstruct the actual course of their distant past history from their words.

Shirley Lindenbaum agrees that, once back beyond living experiences, one is led into the period of mystified history, what the Australian aborigines call the "dream time." Legends and myths, but not real history, are recounted. Yet the two believed that they really were with people for whom the first experience of kuru had indeed occurred in their own lifetimes. Indeed, from the people's verbal testimony they were able to construct a vivid, chronologic account, in which kuru first appeared in the north Fore territory around the turn of the century and then diffused out in an arc into the central-south Fore area. As time passed, sometime in the late 1930s, kuru penetrated farther south in another great arc, eventually reaching Purosa on the southern extremities of the Fore habitations. Lindenbaum explains her belief in the Fore's sense of history this way:

If, in the 1960s, you spoke to people for whom kuru had been a first experience thirty years ago, you had a very strong sense of this chronology. They could tell you all kinds of convincing details – practically what they wore that day, the names of the first people who got the disease in their village, who ate them, to whom they were married, what was going on in their lives at that time, whether they had been initiated, whether they had one or two children. So with hundreds and hundreds of comparable stories we got a sequence of the events and could put the jigsaw together.

By the time the anthropologists left nine months later, their observations had sunk the genetic hypothesis. But they were exhausted. Fieldwork is totally absorbing and must be done for as many hours as necessary, so their breaks from work had been few. Besides being demanding, the experience was also painful, even traumatic. They had shared with the Fore births and moments of joy, bawdy jokes and feasts, but also sadness and deaths, funerals, and bereavements. Worst of all, torn by impotent compassion, they too had watched the Fore experience the hourly agonies of kuru.

Back in Adelaide they made their reports to the Department of Public Health, gave a series of talks, wrote four papers circulated in mimeographed form – one of which presented their data on cannibalism and the possible association with kuru – and attended an informal conference. When Gajdusek was brought in to talk, Shirley Lindenbaum remembers two things vividly: first, the attempt to get him to give a coherent and succinct account of his research. His explosive style was of such torrential force that the Australians could neither contain nor understand him, so they sent him out of the room and gave him twenty-five minutes to organize his thoughts in some sort of sequence. Then he came back and read these slowly, as though to a group of mentally dull children. The second thing she remembers is that the genetic hypothesis for kuru was still such a favorite that their material, with its suggestions of a disease of recent origin and a possible connection with cannibalism, seemed not only exotic but completely out of line. Though Dr. Bennett never contradicted anything they said – indeed, he was very receptive – it was clear that this was not the kind of information he and his colleagues wished to hear. Their data showed that kuru had spread so rapidly in living memory that there was no way a simplistic gene model could accommodate the fact. Still, Glasse and Lindenbaum were encouraged to continue their research and within three months they were back in New Guinea, seeking additional data on a possible correlation between cannibalism and kuru.

The anthropologists returned at a time of crisis. The Fore believed that kuru was the result of malicious sorcery and from that day to this the older people have never seen any reason to change their minds. Their own reputation as sorcerers was fearsome and the appalling evidence before their very eyes – 80 percent of all known cases of kuru occurring in their linguistic group, only 20 percent in their immediate neighbors and none at all beyond – reinforced their belief that their group was under sorcerer's curse. Two hundred people, nearly 1 percent of the Fore, were dying every year. As the death toll rose, particularly among the women, the ratio of adult males to adult females climbed to 2:1; in certain hamlets it reached as high as 3:1. In 1962, nearly half the adult men in Wanitabe had no wives at all and with many children to look after, were forced to assume women's tasks – cooking, weeding, and child rearing. Soon these cultural distortions were reflected in the marriage ceremonies: unless a bride had shown she would survive long enough to produce a child, the bride price would be withheld and the celebratory speeches at the marriage included instructions as to the distribution of the payments should she die.

Kuru was tearing the heart out of the community, the fabric of society was being ripped apart. One afternoon an agitated man from the Yagareba section of the Wanitabe parish stood outside Lindenbaum's house and poured out his agonized thoughts to the people around.

I came here as a boy from the North Fore. I remained here and grew up to lead you in battle after battle. Now my wife has kuru. If someone has caused it, let him remove the poison bundle so she can recover. My legs pain from the distance I have walked searching for cures. During her lifetime she was a woman who looked after the needs of many visitors to our group. She saw they had food and firewood. Now she has kuru. If she dies, there will only be rubbish people left here.

Desperately the Fore searched far and wide for cures. They placed guards on their boundaries to keep out people with malevolent intent. They called openly for confessions of sorcery and where the curse of kuru had been evoked to avenge an insult, propitiations were undertaken. Guilty clans were subject to savage acts of revenge; they were ambushed, stoned, or bitten, and, once again, ritual murders were causing as many deaths as kuru.

At last, in the early sixties, when the Fore faced the specter of extinction, a change suddenly occurred, one borne of total desperation. The unending cycles of fear – the first symptoms, the desperate search for remedies, the inexorable and inevitable personal death, the frantic attempts to avert the tribal fate – reached a climax. Soon there would be no women, and no women meant no children, and no children meant no Fore. Kuru had not been around very long, and earlier periods were clearly far less savage than the present, as revenge, hatred, and murder reached horrendous proportions. In 1962 the *kibungs* took place, gatherings at which people of many different communities came together in what Shirley Lindenbaum describes as an attempt at "moral rearmament of the society"; friendship and unity were stressed; the past as a more golden age remembered; the ancestral myths of their common origins evoked as lodestars to guide the people to a happier future. Drastic changes were coming anyway as the white man moved into the land, so perhaps the moment was ripe for a communal commitment to new ways and better times.

This mood of reconciliation didn't last long. Paradoxically, this had much to do with the white man's belief about kuru. They had told the Fore that kuru was a sickness but, the Fore now realized, this was clearly false. They had similarly told the Fore that yaws was a sickness and *had* cured it, so why did they not cure kuru? And why were mainly women marked and why did no single victim ever recover? Everyone knew sickness was caused by spirits that would catch you if you went into the forest. Yet the chief victims of kuru, the women, rarely went to the forest, and the men who were frequently there rarely got kuru. Sorcery *had* to be the cause.

Although the Fore could not possibly know it, the worst was already over. From now on, kuru would disappear from their midst as mysteriously as it had come. Shirley Lindenbaum would predict this. If the hypothesis she and Robert Glasse now advanced were true, over the years, the number of kuru cases would gradually decline, and there would be no fresh cases except in those people who harbored the disease.

If on their first visit they demolished one hypothesis, on their second they made a major contribution to the mystery of kuru. That they did was, they insist, due to a New Zealander, Dr. R.W. Hornabrook, a neurologist and an epidemiologist, who was doing superb field surveys in the country. "He focused us," Shirley Lindenbaum says, "for he was to ask the right epidemiological question."

Hornabrook looked at their data, immediately perceived a pattern, and set them this task. "Go and find out," he said, "what it is that the adult women and the children of both sexes in the Fore tribe are doing that the adult men are *not* doing. And whatever it is, it is something that the Gimi (an adjacent tribe) are not doing either."

This is precisely what the two anthropologists discovered. By now they were well known in the tribal areas and everywhere made welcome. They lived in the same village and patrolled from time to time, asking questions about kuru and systematically working back to the source of every single piece of information. They had to tread most delicately, for the people were worried that the white men would accuse someone of being the sorcerer behind kuru, and put them in jail, so they were careful to avoid accusations or identifications. Only after a few days settled in one place, would the two begin asking specific questions about kuru: when did it come to your village; where was it before it arrived; who was the first person to catch it; who was the second, the third, and the fourth; what happened to the body? Whenever someone turned up from a distant region they feigned ignorance and went through the whole set of questions again, and gradually they reconfirmed the chronology they had established during their first stay. Now they identified the place, and time, where the first recognizable cases had occurred – in two villages, one in the Fore territory and the other across the border in the Keiagana country. The inhabitants of each accused the others of being the source of kuru.

It was flogging work, day in and day out, questioning, building up the files and cross-checking, while battling against the leeches, avoiding the snakes, and coping with the steamy conditions. Once Glasse had such severe diarrhea that for two days he was blind. Lindenbaum developed a high fever, with tremors and shakes, and for one ghastly moment believed that she was showing first symptoms of the disease she had come to study. They spent hours again tracing kinship patterns, drawing family trees where a *K* marked kuru victims. Most crucial, they drew charts of human flesh-eating, and when they superimposed these on the family trees, they noticed a match between this and the victims of kuru.

Finally they answered Dr. Hornabrook's question and both made contributions. Glasse's was the crystallization of an idea which had been formed during their first visit: he had read an article in *Time* ("Worms, Men and Memory," May 18, 1962) which reported how the memory of simple flatworms was improved by a forced act of cannibalism. In laboratory experiments, ground-up tissue from one worm was fed to another worm which then, it was alleged, acquired the other's memory. True or not, this idea now provided a conceptual framework around which Glasse began to organize their large body of data about cannibalism and kuru.

Lindenbaum's contribution came from her observations of, and her close relationship with, the women. To the question "What is it that the women and the children of the Fore are doing, that the men are not, nor are the people of the Gimi," the answer was, "Sometimes eating each other." Cannibalism, or its associated routines, provided the fourth vital element in the picture, and while not the ultimate cause of kuru it explained the patterns of its attack as first observed by Gajdusek.

As the women freely spoke with Lindenbaum about cannibalism, two extraordinary and quite unexpected facts emerged. First, it was primarily the women who were involved. Second, like kuru, cannibalism was not an ancient tradition but a newly introduced custom that, diffusing in from the north, had not yet penetrated the whole of the Fore. People had been experimenting and there was considerable ambivalence about the practice. There were no rites nor rituals but only a process of "Let's see what it's like." The northern Fore told the anthropologists that around the turn of the century, some elder women, visiting a neighboring tribe to the north that practiced cannibalism, had tried human flesh and found it satisfactory. Over the years the practice gradually diffused south. But now they treated it with high old humor. "Yes — wasn't it funny," they told Lindenbaum, "once we were cannibals."

Like the beginnings of kuru those of cannibalism could be accurately located in historical time. In the extreme south of the Fore area that borders the uninhabited forest, the people remembered the time quite clearly. "It was after the first airplane flew over that we tried cannibalism for the first time." But because most Western people who passed through the area had neither seen cannibalism in action, nor stayed long enough to learn the facts, most of them, Gajdusek included, rejected the anthropologists' hypothesis when they had first heard it.

Why were only the women eating human flesh? Men led largely separate lives and adolescent boys would live in the long houses with the adult men, the hunters, who kept the meat for themselves. The women looked after the pigs but rarely ate them, though the men did. The food of women and small children was mostly vegetables, frogs, insects, or small rodents. The women also prepared the bodies for burial and it was then they occasionally ate part of the flesh. There was no doubt that women, particularly older widows, suffered a lack of protein, and it was these older women who had introduced cannibalistic practices. Indeed, some would deliberately go to funerals, even though not related to the dead person, and join in the wailing and keening, for the deceased was always mourned before being consumed.

When the women laid out the corpses, they would sometimes slice at the flesh with bamboo blades, or pack the brain tissue in small bamboo tubes to be steamed and eaten. Experiments later done at the NIH laboratories showed that more than ten million units of infective kuru agent could be in one gram of such tissue. Still, later experiments, when the animals were given kuru-infected tissue by mouth, showed that inoculation through the skin and mucous membranes was the likely route of infection. Toddlers came to be infected because they played nearby and, from time to time, would be given small pieces to eat. Far more important was the fact that everyone had open sores, or scratches on their skin, so that by handling the dead bodies the majority of the people were probably self-inoculated with the kuru agent passing directly into their bloodstreams.

When in the 1950s cannibalism was forbidden, native constables went from village to village saying, "If you eat people we will *kalabus* you" (jail you). The foreign missionaries, too, hammered home the same message and insisted on proper burial. The total surveillance of kuru which Gajdusek had started, was maintained – by him, by Dr. Michael Alpers, by an Adelaide team, and by government census patrols – and this led to a full registry of all kuru deaths and by 1961 a decline in kuru incidence was evident, with the disease disappearing fast in the youngest age groups. As the practice of cannibalism died down, the incidence of kuru, too, began to fall. Since those years the decline in the incidence of kuru has been unbroken.

Initially most people refused to countenance the anthropologists' theory. It is understandable why Gajdusek initially rejected the idea, because the whole cannibalism connection hinged on the disease being caused by something transmissible – a living organism that passed viably from kuru victim to mourner. But this was still not demonstrated. Moreover, Gajdusek had moved fast through the region, acquiring information as he went, about everything from indigenous music to child rearing to kuru. His facts about the details of cannibalism were at fault: it is clear from his diaries that he thought that the men as well as the women were cannibals. But in that case the much higher incidence in women belied the belief that possible connection between cannibalism and kuru. The anthropologists, staying in one place over a long period, able to penetrate deeper into the matter, could gain a deep understanding of the patterns of Fore life and by now, the answer they gave to Hornabrook's question is one generally accepted. But a good answer always raises another question and this one did: since cannibalism was practiced by many other tribes, why did only the Fore have kuru? So far, this has never been definitively explained, although Gajdusek – and others – have offered several possibilities to explain the appearance of the kuru virus among the Fore.

Finally, in June 1962, the two young people returned to Australia and filed their reports, released their data and distributed another mimeographed paper, "Cannibalism and Kuru." They then moved on to Bangladesh where, in desperate circumstances, they helped in a cholera epidemic and their own partnership foundered. When eight years later Shirley Lindenbaum returned to the Fore, she found the tribe still haunted by kuru and their lives deliberately hidden. In the past all the villages were linked, but now the people blocked off the trails and travelers were kept to the larger roads. The Fore knew that sorcerers were still causing kuru and didn't want any strangers coming through.

Fortunately their blockade didn't last long. As kuru declined, so the Fore began to emerge again and, in any case, other changes were in train. Many young men were leaving to work on the coast or in the lower hill plantations. A money economy entered the Eastern Highlands and the people began producing coffee and other cash crops. By way of compensation for their curse, the Fore had more financial resources pumped into their communities by the government and missionaries than any other groups. Even a hospital was built, which Glasse describes as "positively grandiose" by New Guinea standards. But deep emotional scars remained on all – Fore and foreigners alike.

By 1963, too, the epidemiological profile of kuru and its pattern of attack were established and explained. Kuru had first appeared exclusively among those women who had tried human flesh for the first time. They have all long since died. Then came a battalion of childhood and adolescent cases as well, with the sexes equally at risk, consisting of those boys and girls who, as the toddlers, had played around the adult women as the latter performed their tasks. They, too, have all died. After a further period, during which cannibalism was totally proscribed, childhood and adolescent cases disappeared completely. By 1970 there were only two twelve-year-old patients; by May 1978, the youngest patient was twenty years old and today no childhood or adolescent cases exist. The only people still left with kuru are some twenty adults who, as toddlers, had played near their mothers during the last years before cannibalism disappeared, and in whom the infection took a very long time to emerge. Soon they too will be dead and kuru will have vanished forever.

1963 was a crisis year for the Fore, for they faced extinction. It was a crucial year for Robert Glasse and Shirley Lindenbaum, as they completed their studies and their personal partnership dissolved. It was crucial for Carleton Gajdusek and Joe Gibbs too, because they began to inject chimpanzees with brain tisue. But in 1963 Joe Smadel died, still believing that, one day, the golden positive would finally turn up. Soon it did. Two years after Smadel's death Joe Gibbs was in southern France

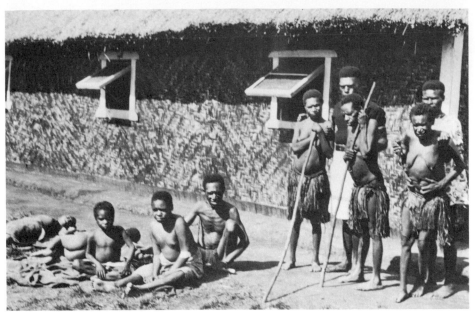

Three adult female kuru patients standing before the Pintogori Kuru Hospital supported by native medical assistants, and five children seated in front. All patients had died of kuru within one year after photograph had been taken.
(D. Carleton Gajdusek)

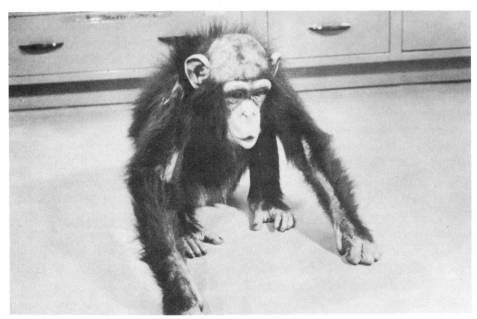

Georgette, the first chimpanzee to show signs of kuru, here demonstrates the unsteady posture and vacant stare typical of kuru. (D. Carleton Gajdusek)

attending a meeting on scrapie and presenting a paper expounding the hypothesis that kuru was probably an infectious, and therefore, a transmissible disease. Arriving in the States, he was called to the telephone, to be alerted to an odd change in one of the chimpanzees. Without even unpacking he drove straight to Patuxent to examine Georgette, who twenty months earlier had been inoculated with a suspension of frozen brain material from a kuru patient. She was shaking with typical kuru tremors. Daisy, another chimpanzee, was also ill, and both had the characteristic blank, withdrawn expression of the kuru victim. Staring, amazed, Gibbs saw the human disease mirrored in these animals. It was so incredible, he now says, that he couldn't believe what he was seeing. Gajdusek was out of the country; Gibbs was in charge and wasn't sure what to do next. For a couple of weeks the group watched the disease progress into its terminal stages, and then decided to sacrifice the animal.

They flew in one of their closest collaborators, Dr. Elisabeth Beck, a neuropathologist from England. Four people from the Armed Forces Institute of Pathology also came to help. The autopsy they carried out was in stark contrast to those Gajdusek had performed in New Guinea. A meticulously clean and sterile area was established in the cold, bleak laboratory, for they could not risk introducing into the animal's tissues any agent not previously there. There had to be no ambiguity: the sterile field had to be scrupulously maintained, for whatever the disease, it had to be shown to be a total response to that one inoculation of human kuru material, placed in Georgette two years before.

Gowned, masked, and gloved, the scientists cut through the chimpanzee skull and removed the brain gently, careful not to distort the tissue. In the next room Elisabeth Beck, gowned, masked, and gloved, packed the brain with utmost care, to take back with her to her own laboratory in England. Soon she was on the transatlantic telephone with her preliminary report: the pathological lesions were some of the most striking and rapid she had ever seen and totally consistent with a kuru infection.

Suddenly, the other chimpanzee, Daisy, died, then Hermann, then George. Gajdusek, visiting Australia, was on the telephone in a constant frenzy: "Send a brain here, send another there" till Gibbs worried they would run out. But, now he says simply, "Thank God, we didn't. And soon we had all the evidence to prove that we had transmitted kuru. It was the first degenerative disease of the human central nervous system that had been shown to be caused by a transmissible infectious agent. The clinical signs in the animals mimicked the disease we had seen in humans; the pathology too, was almost exactly the same."

Their excitement intensified when the full report came from Elisabeth Beck. The most striking pathological feature was the extensive, spongy degeneration of the tissue, with so many holes that, under the microscope, the sections looked like pieces of Swiss cheese. This information was as electrifying as earlier Bill Hadlow's idea had been, because suddenly the group remembered that, six years before, Igor Klatzo had drawn attention to the similarity of kuru with Creutzfeldt-Jakob disease, CJD, another condition in which brain sections look like Swiss cheese. Klatzo, too, now examined their chimpanzee brain sections, and besides holes there were plaques, that seemed identical with those he had seen before, both in kuru victims and in known CJD cases. The conclusion was inescapable: kuru wasn't a unique disease and there was another one like it much closer to home.

Immediately the group searched for a brain from a Creutzfeldt-Jakob patient and finally they did find one of spongiform encephalopathy, a descriptive name that simply means a brain with a lot of holes in it. Elisabeth Beck sent them this sample from England and, in 1968, a chimpanzee was inoculated with it. In less than one year, a shorter time than had ever been the case with kuru, the animal died with clinical symptoms and pathological lesions, similar to kuru and CJD. This particular result electrified Western medicine, for it revealed that the scientists were dealing, not with an exotic disease in a remote population that most physicians in the world would never see, but with a medical problem that, though rare, had been described in Western populations. This, Gibbs insists, was even more exciting than their experimental transmission of kuru because it meant that Gajdusek's prediction which had kept him and his colleagues grappling with the mysterious disease of New Guinea for years was coming true: kuru had great significance for other neurodegenerative diseases. Within just two years the group collected some three or four hundred cases of such diseases, from neurological and neurosurgical clinics throughout the world, and it was constantly seeing the white holes and the famous plaques.

By 1968, the NIH group definitely proved that two degenerative diseases of the human central nervous system were caused by a filterable infective agent which, from first exposure, had a minimum incubation period of about a year and often much longer. Infection it might be, yet it produced none of the inflammatory pathology characteristic of typical brain infections. Illnesses with this quite extraordinary pattern were striking newcomers onto the human medical scene – and slow viruses were their cause.

The consequences were equally dramatic: one was Gajdusek's Nobel Prize in 1976. He took along eight of his adopted Micronesian and Melanesian sons to the ceremony in Stockholm and made one of his rare appearances on television. Other consequences were more practical but equally startling. Medicine was now facing diseases provoked by agents so different from normal viruses that the sterilization techniques *in every operating room on earth* had to change, even those in dentistry. Techniques that, up to this moment, were thought to be adequate for sterilization of instruments, proved to be useless against slow viruses so the very latest ethylene oxide sterilizers, then used in every operating room, were discarded and old-fashioned ones restored. Extra money had to be spent on different methods of autoclaving. Shortcuts to sterilization which had been adopted, using noncorrosive antiseptics, were found not to work at all.

Unexplained deaths in neuroscience now began to make sense. All patients who develop neurologic disorders of this type die of progressive, severe disease. There are *no* exceptions. Then, appallingly, some classic viruses were shown to be able to switch behavior: the common measles virus, which normally produces a self-limiting disease, goes underground in a few unlucky children and one to twenty years later produces a chronic degenerative neurologic illness that kills the young adult.

Suddenly, scientists all over the world began searching for slow viruses everywhere, wondering whether diseases such as amyotrophic lateral sclerosis, Alzheimer's, multiple sclerosis, osteoarthritis, diabetes, and even schizophrenia might all be due to similar lurking viruses. When researchers looked for such viruses, they often found them, even in the most unexpected places. One disease, progressive multifocal leukoencephalopathy, is caused by a slow virus that most of us have in our brains right now, and most will die without ever knowing it. But in a very few, unlucky people, whose immune system has been suppressed by cancer treatment or by immunosuppressive procedures following an organ transplant, the virus sometimes becomes alive and a fatal brain disease follows.

Thus, far from being the end of the story, the solution of the kuru mystery was just the beginning. Starting with an obscure disease in a Stone Age tribe, scientists had uncovered a whole group of rare disorders caused by chronic slow virus infections, and, to their amazement, the first one they had stumbled on was mirrored in a presenile dementia, Creutzfeldt-Jakob disease, found everywhere. Then another possibility occurred

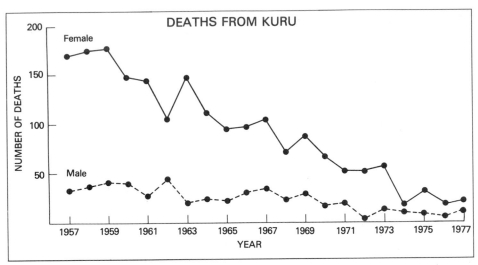

The overall incidence of kuru deaths in male and female patients by year since its discovery in 1957 through 1977. More than 2,500 patients died of kuru during this 20-year period of surveillance. The decline in incidence of the disease followed the cessation of cannibalism, which occurred between 1957 and 1962 in various villages. (D. Carleton Gajdusek)

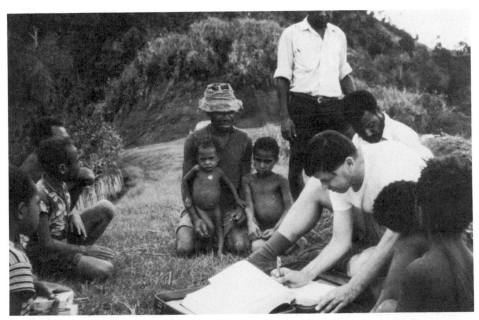

Dr. Gajdusek at work in the Anga (Kukukuku) region of New Guinea in 1972, surrounded by his usual crowd. (D. Carleton Gajdusek; archive # IGM-72-NG-18-21)

to them, triggered by Gajdusek's 1957 likening of kuru to a "galloping senesence of juveniles." Kuru and CJD were dementias acquired in early or middle age. Yet was it possible that the senile dementias – those disorders of old age – were similarly caused, a consequence not so much of the passage of time but of slow infections?

Was it ever possible perhaps that grandparents could transmit a slow virus infection to grandchildren? There is complete agreement on the answer to that question: a categorical "There is no risk whatever," for we must distinguish between infections and contagions. Slow viruses certainly can somehow insinuate themselves deep into the genetic apparatus of cells and indeed may have been acquired during the course of evolution. But drastic cultural patterns as in kuru, or accidents as in brain surgery, are necessary to pass them from person to person as infections. Direct communicability from simple contact does not occur. Nevertheless, though these viruses are not contagious they can be inherited. One familial form of CJD has been traced back to 1840, in one family's tree. This special form of CJD is called Gerstmann-Straussler syndrome (GSS), and in this family did not miss a single line: only a few family members in any one generation came through unscathed. In such families the disease behaves as though it were caused by a single Mendelian dominant gene. Yet even so, Gajdusek's group at NIH and an independent British team transmitted this disease horizontally by inoculating primates with the brain tissue of GSS patients.

This was yet another incredible result in a continuingly incredible story, for it ran counter to accepted opinion, which said that genetic diseases were one thing, but viral diseases were utterly distinct. But the experimental facts are compelling and though certain dementias *are* genetic familial diseases, that may have run through many generations, it is still possible that a virus causes them and that it can be transmitted.

Once again the consequences have been dramatic. Scientists researching classical genetic diseases, like the familial type of Alzheimer's disease, Pick's disease, and Huntington's Chorea, now put a significant part of their budgets and effort searching for a virus, possibly lurking behind the genetic defect, while those scientists specializing in slow-virus diseases are searching for an underlying genetic cause. How does the heredity apparatus connect with these slow viruses? This fundamental question encompasses one of the greatest challenges in contemporary science, for even though a slow virus may not be contagious, it clearly can insinuate itself, not only into the brain but into the genetic apparatus too, and be inherited. Cancer biologists think that certain specific cancer-causing genes may have a similar viral origin.

But whether or not it is the cause of dementias or cancers, the virus hides. It replicates in only part and, for some reason, the body's immune system totally fails to respond. Just what the virus actually does in the brain, and why, and how this leads to the neural shambles of Swiss cheese, and, in some cases, amyloid plaques, we still have no idea. How these pathological changes are triggered remains a mystery of great concern to scientists and to clinicians.

The challenges posed by slow viruses and their diseases rival even those of cancer in complexity, consequences, and in the sheer difficulty of finding effective remedies. If scientists are to make an impact on their diseases they will have to gain a comprehensive understanding of them, as Gajdusek did with kuru, trying to find the agent that causes them and how its structure provokes the pathological damage doctors finally see. Contemporary scientists do, of course, have a great advantage because they now have more sophisticated biochemical tools than when Gajdusek began work thirty years ago. But the deeper they probe the more complex the problems seem.

For a start, the brain tissue and structure of these dementias reveal the end result of pathological damage, not the causes. Looking at damaged nerve cells in a dead person and speculating what might have occurred twenty years before is like looking at a burnt-out star and speculating what might have occurred millions of years before. The lesions in the brain do not reveal when the disease started, nor how, nor the structure of the infectious agent, nor what biochemical changes it first provoked that ultimately led to the neuronal shambles that eventually kills. Brain biopsies are sometimes done in dementia patients to establish the diagnosis, and they can reveal some of the changes that precede death. But for experimental study of the disease, an animal model must be created: scientists must try to reproduce the disease in the laboratory and to trace its progression. To do this, scientists want to be able to inoculate their animals, not with crude suspension of diseased human tissue, but rather a purified and concentrated suspension of the slow virus in question. Only then can they expect to understand the biochemical nature of these mysterious holes that appear in the brain.

So far no scientist can say, with any confidence, that a slow virus – or indeed a part of it – has been detected by electron microscopy. Some scientists have claimed to have done so, and they have been looking for the particle in a very familiar place – in the plaques of the damaged brain.

For these strange, beautiful structures, which in numbers and distribution are directly correlated to the severity of the person's dementia, provide the focus for investigation and debate. In kuru, or CJD, or senile dementias, or just an aged brain, plaques are present and the correlation is exquisitely simple. We will all have plaques in our brains eventually if we live long enough. The older we are, no matter who we are, the more there will be. The more there are, the greater the loss of memory and intellect, and the greater the destruction of the personality. In the dementias associated with slow viruses the plaques increase in number and distribution for reasons we don't yet understand.

The functional effect of a plaque is easy enough to understand, for it is so solid a structure that nerve cells cannot communicate across it. Consequently the highways and freeways of the brain – the neuronal axons – get jammed, and the carriers of the messages – whether chemical or electrical – can no longer move, for the axons of the nerve cells no longer transmit nerve impulses. Thus, interference with axonal transport is, Gajdusek believes, the problem on which to focus. The question is this: are these plaques merely a late consequence of a disease process that began many years earlier, or, if slow viruses are the root cause of the trouble, are the plaques themselves the cause of the disease?

Some scientists, Gajdusek included, believe that there are many specific ways, viral and nonviral, to block the flow down the nerve axon and the important challenge is to find ways to unblock the traffic jam, and get the whole system moving again. There is no longer the same urgency to concentrate on the many specific causes.

Other scientists, however, are as obsessed by the challenge of the cause, as Gajdusek had been with kuru, and are confident that the structural and functional mysteries of these dementias lie in the plaques as surely as the mysteries of kuru did in the brain. Piquantly, once more, scientists in this search have returned to scrapie and the plaques it provokes. One has a paradoxical situation in that at the New York State Institute for Basic Research in Developmental Disabilities on Staten Island (directed by Dr. Henry M. Wisniewski), scientists working on the senile dementia, Alzheimer's disease, are focusing on this disease of sheep. And the very first question they attempted to answer was the one we have just defined: are scrapie plaques clumps of slow viruses, or merely the damage that the viruses cause?

Those who study scrapie start with a built-in advantage because it can be easily transmitted to laboratory mice. So the progressive stages in the dementia can be described and the progressive development of the plaques at all stages uncovered. They consist of a protein, called amyloid: no matter where plaques come from — whether CJD patients, or scrapie sheep, or Alzheimer patients — there is this protein. Patricia Merz, an electron microscopist, was given the job of searching for the slow viruses behind scrapie. In her quest Merz followed the good, old-fashioned routines of observation — sectioning the brain, staining the slides, and taking photographs through her electron microscope — very much as Klatzo had done years before — and one day stumbled on something she had never seen before.

Over and over again, she saw long thin fibrils in the diseased sections of scrapie brain, whether from hamsters or mice. She found them in different strains of scrapie, trying five in all. The fibrils could be seen in the animals long before the first clinical symptoms appeared; they increased in numbers as incubation continued. Their shape was completely unlike any animal virus ever seen before, though they reminded scientists of the filamentous viruses that attack plants and bacteria.

The same question asked about plaques had to be asked about fibrils. Were these fibrils caused by scrapie or are they the cause of scrapie? Over a painstaking year, with the systematic urgency of a detective on a murderer's trail, Dr. Merz built up a photographic dossier on the fibrils. She found them in a wide range of animals and under a range of conditions. She did not find them in mice that were merely aged, but she did find them in mice, hamsters, and squirrel monkeys, that had been inoculated with scrapie. She found them also in brain extracts from CJD patients, in brains from kuru patients, in animals with experimentally induced CJD, and in experimentally induced kuru. She did not find them in Parkinson's disease, nor in Alzheimer's disease, nor in the brains from human controls.

The evidence at this stage is quite insufficient to say whether or not these fibrils are the virus. All Merz will now say is that there is a good correlation between their presence and the diseases caused by unconventional slow viruses. Hedging her bets, as Gajdusek had hedged his, she says that she is looking at either the result of the disease process, or the actual slow virus, or a component of it. This is a suitably cautious and open conclusion. Yet, it must be emphasized that, in the years since her work began, scrapie-associated fibrils have been exclusively observed in unconventional slow virus diseases and *nowhere else*. The exciting fact is that, unlike the holes, the tangles, and the plaques, these fibrils are being seen *long before* the clinical symptoms appear, and in organs that are subsequently unaffected by the disease and where no damage results.

Therefore, Pat Merz concludes, that it is quite likely they are the cause of the problem.

All this is a long way from proof, of course, and though the number of scientists working on this problem is still small, the Staten Island scientists do face much competition, from scientists like Stanley Prusiner in San Francisco. Though there is much debate and even dissension over some of the claims being made, there is general agreement that a Nobel Prize awaits the scientist who finally does identify the structure of the slow virus.

Behind all this science the human victims stand. The agonies these dementias provoke can be as devastating to the families as kuru was to the Fore. Who are the people who are catching these diseases and what is the dimension of the problems we are facing?

Janet, forty-nine years old, the mother of three grown-up children, lives in Weybridge, Surrey, Great Britain, and has the fatal brain dementia, the GSS form of CJD. Whereas kuru attacks the cerebellar centers that control muscular coordination, GSS destroys the cerebral parts of the brain responsible for the intellect. When, a few years ago, the symptoms first appeared, Janet's husband, Len, knew that after thirty years of marriage life was coming to an end. He has taken on tasks previously assumed by his wife – vacuuming, shopping, cooking, mending – combining his own work as an electrician with the roles of nurse and housekeeper. Communication is difficult: though Janet does know Len and her children, and can remember some things from the distant past, her memory of immediate events, such as what she had for breakfast ten minutes before, has totally disappeared. Wonderfully healthy, vibrantly alive with the happiest of smiles, Janet appears at first glance to be a normal woman, but a short time in her company reveals a lost mind imprisoned in an active body.

It was Len who tracked the presenile dementia through Janet's family tree for one hundred and forty years, finding that GSS had been a constant curse. Though the pattern is not entirely predictable, Len knows that his children may be affected, for no single generation where the mother had GSS was missed. It was a sample of brain from Janet's second cousin, who also died of GSS, that British scientists injected into a marmoset monkey, so demonstrating that this dementia could be transmitted horizontally, as well as inherited vertically, down through the generations.

Fortunately, presenile dementias, like CJD and its variant, GSS, are rare. More people are killed in traffic accidents every day than from

CJD in one year, and some will survive while the three hundred Americans who die of CJD every year never have a chance.

By contrast senile dementias are not rare at all and the most common is Alzheimer's disease, whose numbers are now causing serious concern. There is still much controversy over whether or not Alzheimer's disease is caused by a slow virus. Gajdusek had once speculated that it might be, but now (1985) he is convinced that it is not. Certainly there may be biochemical similarities in the brain plaques of CJD patients, Alzheimer patients, kuru patients, and animals with scrapie. But the hallmarks of these dementias – the great vacuoles – are not present in the pathology of the Alzheimer brain; nor has the disease ever been transmitted to animals by experimental inoculation. What similarities do exist between all these dementias may result from nerve damage blocking the neural pathways.

Whatever the cause of Alzheimer's disease, the human effects are devastating. Jim Lube, fifty-three years old, lives in San Francisco. His wife is Japanese and they have two children. Jim worked at the check-out counter in the local supermarket for he was a wizard at the cash register until gradually he began to make errors, yet was unaware he was making them. Slowly it became clear that he had Alzheimer's disease. He became more and more confused and forgetful; his estimates of time or distance or place were soon totally obscured. The pattern of profound mental retardation was typical: the higher functions erode first as memory goes, then intellect, then finally personality and awareness. So now the family has to care for their father as if he were a child.

Says Karen, his daughter,

We found out two years ago that Dad had Alzheimer's disease, when he suddenly had a lot of complications at work. Now it's really hard to remember what he was like before. He's two different people. It's my father but my Dad has gone. It's really a terrible thing to say, but it's like he's losing all his human qualities. There's a lot of regression, confusion, and anger and I think that he feels enough to realize that he doesn't understand what's happening. Right now it's just not possible for us to have Dad taken care of professionally. We did have him in a day care program, but the state funding was cut off, so he's not able to go there now. He's not yet bad enough to need twenty-four hour care, but he will soon, and then I don't quite know what's going to happen. The doctors say that it's quite possible for him to hang on for a decade, just slowly getting worse each month and year. I can't imagine what it's going to be like when he is not able to talk, and that's the scariest part. Alzheimer's is such a selfish disease. It goes so slow and takes everything away.

The statistics of Alzheimer's disease show that it truly deserves the label "epidemic" and one comes to see why, in terms of personal distress and social disruption, this problem may well be the kuru of our society. Twenty-five million people in the United States aged sixty-five or older now have Alzheimer's disease. Ten percent of the population – that is, 2.5 million people – are mildly or moderately demented from it; 5 percent (1.3 million people) require institutionalization. Presently 56 percent of all beds in nursing homes are occupied by the demented, and they can survive for years. The financial and emotional burdens on families and society are enormous and the problem is going to grow much worse because the numbers at risk, in the United States alone, will double to fifty million in the next sixty years, as the baby boom generation becomes "senior citizens."

It was only a few generations ago, we thought that as we grew older we would naturally become more absentminded and dotty simply because we *were* getting old. But now doctors know it's not that simple. They suspect that all dementias might be infections that can develop if you live long enough, and in the West we mostly do.

Thus, the story that began far away from the civilization most of us inhabit, with the search for the cause of a disease in an obscure Stone Age tribe, has led remorselessly to the diseases that may devastate us all. For young scientists, who love the mystery of complex problems, there is no greater challenge than that posed by the problems of slow viruses and the mechanisms that cause neurologic diseases. But there is no way the results or the therapies can come quickly, both because the problems are so difficult and because, as Dr. Lewis Thomas recently wrote in a poignant essay on dementias, it takes so long before even the most tentative of findings can emerge. Even the most obsessed of scientists, who revel in intriguing and engrossing problems, tend to stay away from long-term puzzles. Perhaps what Lewis Thomas was implying is that there aren't enough Gajduseks around; perhaps there are too few flamboyant, obsessed people, prepared to gamble and devote a quarter century to results that may never arrive, and too few people like Joe Smadel, another man who was willing to gamble. If this is true, then Joe Smadel will be turning in his grave for the golden days of American science will have vanished. And, if this is true, then we in Western society will be perpetually cursed with the problem of dementias, as surely as the Fore might, so easily, have been perpetually cursed with the plague of the sorcerers – until their tribe had gone.

2
Vaccine on Trial

The wounded surgeon plies the steel
That questions the distempered part;
Beneath the bleeding hands we feel
The sharp compassion of the healer's art
Resolving the enigma of the fever chart.

T. S. Eliot, "East Coker," Four Quartets

Gay men were aware that they faced some special health problems even before Wolf Szmuness appeared in their lives. These did not appear as sudden epidemics, as acquired immune deficiency syndrome (AIDS) did a decade later, but crept in slowly and remorselessly. The men suspected that their sexual habits were part of the problem but, in the early 1970s, were not ready to change their life-style. These were the heady days of a gay liberation movement that began in 1969, when a police raid on a homosexual bar in Christopher Street, New York, provoked a riot by its patrons. The street and its vicinity in Greenwich Village became a focus of gay activity. Here in the bars or just on the streets, homosexuals could find friends and mentors, casual contacts or steady lovers, the possibility of a devoted, lasting relationship or a transient, anonymous promiscuity. At weekends or on "buddy" nights, five hundred to one thousand men might gather in the bathhouses, where a man could make several random sexual contacts in the course of one evening – by the 1970s the police raids had stopped.

Along with liberation came an increase in certain diseases: syphilis, gonorrhea, and hepatitis B were the most serious. By 1972 gay men were so concerned about these and the quality of health care available through orthodox channels, that they organized the Gay Men's Health Project. Started by Len Ebreo, staffed by a physician, Dr. Daniel William, together with male nurses and volunteers, financed by voluntary donations and the Bureau of Venereal Disease Control in New York City, the Project's activities rapidly expanded. Screening for venereal disease was offered first and was so effective that soon the Project was discovering higher levels of asymptomatic syphilis and gonorrhea than the other comparable screening programs in New York City.

If the familiar sexually transmitted diseases were a serious problem, it rapidly became clear that hepatitis B was far worse. It was once believed that, as a viral disease, it could only be contracted via a contaminated needle or the blood of an infectious donor. But a crucial series of experiments by Dr. Saul Krugman in the 1960s showed that hepatitis B *is* infectious and can spread from person to person by contact and sexual intimacy. It had been suspected in the years since that discovery that gay men had a higher prevalence of this disease than other, comparable groups. When a physician saw an adult male in his twenties with acute hepatitis B, the first inference was that he was either a drug addict or a homosexual.

Each year 200,000 new cases of hepatitis B occur in the United States; 52,000 show signs of liver damage, 10,000 will be hospitalized; and 250 people will die of acute fulminating liver failure. The symptoms range from very mild to totally disabling. The first ones are as mild as those of a slight cold. But the illness can build into a condition so debilitating that patients may sleep twenty hours a day and cannot take care of themselves. Since they can function for only two to three hours at a time and can never tell in advance which these will be, they must give up work, social activities, and inevitably most friendships. This pattern is common to all who contract hepatitis B, and, psychologically, its consequences can be devastating.

There is no treatment, but since the vast majority have only mild disease, with adequate rest and a liver not assaulted with alcohol, the body's defense systems can cope and patients make a full recovery. Others have persistent liver inflammation, and a small percentage of these go on to develop chronic liver disease. In yet others the speed of attack is so quick that the immune system is overwhelmed and death rapidly follows from fulminating liver failure.

Unhappily, the problems are not confined to those who catch hepatitis B. Acute cases *may* be rare, but unfortunately the virus is a silent killer and a high proportion of its victims never clear it from their blood. So not only do they have a permanent, debilitating condition but they are "carriers" and thus sources of infection. There are thousands of carriers in the United States, and each year the numbers increase by 3 percent.

Hepatitis B is not just a serious problem for gay men in Western society. It poses one of the greatest problems for global public health, the major endemic areas being Asia and Africa, especially below the Sahara.

Several hundred thousand carriers may be walking around the United States, but in the areas where the disease is endemic there are ten million. Two hundred million people have an active infection. Many develop chronic liver disease and between one to two million are acutely ill. A further five to seven million people are at risk, and the consequences are nasty, for scientific studies have revealed overwhelming evidence of a clear-cut connection between hepatitis B and liver cancer. Doctors can say, convincingly, that hepatitis B virus is probably *the* major cause of liver cancer anywhere. If you contract hepatitis B, it doesn't mean you will get liver cancer; but if you have liver cancer, you certainly once had an attack of hepatitis B. A chronic carrier has a 270 times greater chance of contracting liver cancer than other people. The earlier in life the infection is contracted, the greater this risk. In those countries where health standards are low and the pool of infection is constantly being replaced as mothers transmit the virus to newborn children, the statistics mirror this fact. Thus in Africa every second cancer patient, whether male or female, has liver cancer; in both Africa and Asia liver cancer is the primary cancer killer of all men between the ages of twenty-five and thirty; in Asia, most especially China, it is the second major cancer in *all* groups. Thus any remedy for hepatitis B would reduce the incidence of one of the world's worst, and most widespread, cancers.

Though these facts would in time greatly influence the way in which gay men regarded hepatitis B and the steps they would take to eliminate it, to begin with, they were totally unaware of the global implications. In fact they were woefully ignorant of its dimensions even within their own community. They knew only that it was their major medical problem even though it wasn't clear which of the four types of hepatitis gay men were mostly contracting, nor how any of the hepatitis was being transmitted. Soon they were deeply troubled and not only about their own health problems, but also about their image. To be gay in the early 1970s meant more than just practicing the sex life of one's choice. There was a sense that one should be politically active too, and contribute not only to the gay rights movement but also to the wider public good. So when in 1973 the Gay Men's Health Project was approached by Mr. Isaac Much, assistant to Dr. Wolf Szmuness at the Laboratory of Epidemiology at the New York Blood Center, and asked to participate in a hepatitis study, the group readily agreed. The study was part of a large national survey to determine the prevalence of hepatitis in a variety of populations, including Chinese-Americans, blood donors, and medical personnel as well as gay men. Under the aegis of the Gay Men's Health Project four hundred young homosexuals supplied blood samples and answered a detailed, and very intimate questionnaire about their sexual history and private lives.

Fortunately, by then, the hepatitis B virus could be conclusively identified in blood by virtue of a specific protein molecule that it produces on its surface and uses to latch onto the liver cells. This protein is also the molecule to which the defending immune system of the body responds, by producing antibodies that smother it and so prevent the virus penetrating the liver cells. It is the presence in the blood of both these antibodies and traces of this viral protein, the flecks from the virus's overcoat, that reveal whether a person has acquired a protective immunity to hepatitis B or is a carrier and still harboring the virus.

The results of the study were far worse than anyone had suspected, and the gay community was shaken. Whereas only 5 percent of the general adult population showed a prior exposure to hepatitis B – with people from the poorer sections of society and recently arrived immigrants from underdeveloped countries predominating – more than 50 percent of the gay community showed evidence of the disease. The chances of a sexually active, urban homosexual male being infected with hepatitis B were better than 1 in 2, and the greater the number of different sexual contacts he had, the higher this risk. An active male homosexual was ten to fifteen times more likely to contract the disease than an active male heterosexual; the chances were better than 2 in 3 and this figure still stands. Of the 200,000 new cases that occur of hepatitis B in any one year in America, gay men form by far the highest portion. Each year 12 percent of the gay population afresh contract the disease.

The study revealed several other facts. A patient with the disease could be infectious for months, even years, and the virus spread rapidly during close contact. Even the smallest drop of blood was dangerous and could transmit the disease through the minutest break in the body's surface membranes. Hepatitis B particles were found in saliva, in semen, and in urine. Given these facts, it became obvious how hepatitis B came to be a problem for gay men.

The prospects were grim. There was no treatment, no cure, no prevention, and no protection. For though the virus had been characterized, no one had succeeded in culturing it – the first step toward making a vaccine. So, far worse than venereal diseases, which did at least respond to antibiotics, hepatitis B threatened to become a curse of the gay community. The men well knew that those who took moralistic attitudes toward them would consider this curse well deserved. Liberated as they may have been, they still felt alienated.

Yet, ironically, it would be through hepatitis B that the gay community of Greenwich Village, New York, made a major contribution to the health of all nations. And piquantly, the man who provided this opportunity was an alien of another kind. In late middle age, his career in ruins and his life shipwrecked, he had been tossed up on the shores of the New World by the unpredictable tide of fortune.

One afternoon in the spring of 1969, the director of the New York Blood Center, Dr. Aaron Kellner, took a telephone call from an old friend, Dr. Walsh McDermott, professor and chairman of the Department of Public Health at Cornell University Medical Center, just a couple of blocks away on the upper East Side. McDermott came straight to the point: an odd little man – a Dr. Wolf Szmuness – had just turned up who said he was a physician-epidemiologist with a special interest in hepatitis. He had produced a number of published scientific papers, but they were all in Polish or Russian and McDermott understood neither language. The stranger was desperate for a job; did the Blood Center have any openings? Kellner recalls,

I didn't know that we had a job for an epidemiologist, but I did know that we were interested in epidemiology as a possibility for a laboratory. I had long felt that a blood center is an ideal milieu for an epidemiologist, with a gold mine of material, but we had no specific budget line for any such position. However, I asked Walsh to call Dr. Fred Prince, the head of our virology laboratory, who specialized in hepatitis, to see if he had openings. All that Fred had was the very lowest possible position of laboratory technician, yet when this was offered to Dr. Szmuness he accepted it instantly – almost hungrily. So a few days later he joined our staff as "Research Associate" with a small salary and a very menial job helping the investigators do various procedures, a range of blood tests and the like.

When I first laid eyes on Wolf Szmuness my heart sank. I saw a short, timid man with a large head, deeply pockmarked face and a vivid shock of thick yellow hair, shabbily dressed in threadbare clothes. He rarely looked anyone in the eye; his gaze was always riveted to the ground. He walked huddled close to the wall as if he were afraid of being struck. All in all he presented a picture of a thoroughly cowed and beaten man, a pathetic figure. I didn't appreciate that this was going to be even much of a technician, much less an epidemiologist. What I couldn't tell, of course, at that time, was that within him lay the seeds of genius.

Over the next few years the story of Szmuness's life gradually emerged. He came from a middle-class Jewish family in Warsaw, Poland.

In 1937, when he was eighteen, he went to the University of Pisa, Italy, to study medicine and in September, 1939 came home for vacation. But that was the month when the German armies invaded Poland, so unable to return to Italy Szmuness enrolled at the University of Lublin. When Stalin and Hitler divided Poland, many Poles faced a crucial decision: to stay or to go. Szmuness sped back to Warsaw to persuade his parents to accompany him to the Russian sector. But they were as frightened of the Russians as he was of the Germans. His parents vanished in the Holocaust; Szmuness finished up in Siberia.

There was little time to spend on persuasion, for the German armies were moving fast. With his friend Pavel, he fled southeast, back to Lublin where a temporary border point was open. They crossed the frontier and eventually came to a small town in the Urals near the Volga River, in the state of Bashkirskaya, where Szmuness was sent to help control the recurring outbreaks of disease. He had wanted to go and fight Hitler at the front, but being both a Jew and a foreigner he was a natural focus of suspicion. Eventually the authorities said he could join the "internal army" and sent him to Siberia.

On December 3, 1942, he, with many others, was moved hundreds of miles east, to a special labor camp near the small town of Prokop'yevsk. This was not a prison as such; he could live in the town but was forbidden to leave the area. Here began a long dark period, toiling underground in the mines and at hard labor in the forests. Intense physical effort on minuscule rations and unsanitary conditions provoked dreadful medical problems. Along with local Russians and fellow prisoners, Szmuness suffered badly from tuberculosis and malnutrition, exacerbated by the grinding work and penetrating cold. His feet, too swollen to take shoes, were wrapped in rags and paper. Had life gone on like that he would have soon died. But some of his comrades, aware that diseases were rapidly spreading, spoke to the authorities. They wanted this "naïve" doctor to look after the cafeteria, check the food, and maintain the general health of the camp. So, one day, without a word of explanation, he was reassigned.

His medical techniques were, of course, extremely basic – controlling outbreaks of lice, diagnosing disease, isolating infectious people, and generally looking after the sanitation. The local doctors soon discovered that he was very clever; he was given more important jobs, better rations, and eventually was made "chief of epidemiology" in the little town. He remained in the camp for two years, but even after he was let out he had to stay in Siberia. In all he spent fifteen and a half years in "internal exile." During that time he finished his medical studies, met his wife, and decided on his area of research.

He completed his medical degree at the University of Tomsk shortly before he met his future wife, Maya, in May 1946. Her father was a doctor practicing in a small country town where Szmuness was sent to help control an epidemic of typhoid fever. "The first time we met," she says, "he didn't pay to me any attention. Then one evening my father and Wolf finished in the hospital early and came back for dinner. Afterward we stayed up and talked and talked. Wolf swore he would never marry because it would be silly to abandon his duty in such difficult times. I said I would not marry either, for the same reason. He decided to marry me one week later."

If being assigned to public health duties at the camp was his first stroke of good fortune, marrying Maya was his second. In the partnership of thirty-six years that followed, it was her decisiveness, confidence, realism, practicality that released a flood of creativity in Wolf Szmuness. He would remain impractical, innocently trusting, and nervously fearful.

His fears were perfectly rational though, for during the Stalinist purges he had been interrogated several times and told to spy on his colleagues, reveal "plots" and expose "traitors." In spite of several beatings and a battery of psychological and physical assaults he refused to cooperate. Finally they gave up but one day, in an interview that would haunt him always, a KGB agent pointed "a long finger" at him and said: "Say nothing of this to anyone, but remember. We will reach you anywhere in the world. No matter where you go, no matter where you try to hide, you will never be out of our grasp."

Sometimes he thought of returning to Poland, but he was too afraid and, anyway, was happy enough with the life that he could now live with his wife and their small daughter, Helena, whom he adored. When he was finally allowed to leave Siberia, the family went to Char'kov in the Ukraine. Here he took an advanced scientific degree, equivalent to the Ph.D., at the university and in 1955 he became chief of the Department of Epidemiology at the Institute for Postgraduate Physicians, at Zoporozh'ye, also in the Ukraine. At this time Maya Szmuness developed hepatitis after a postoperative blood transfusion, and nearly died. Wolf Szmuness was to spend the next twenty-three years exclusively studying the patterns of this disease.

In 1959, twenty years after he had first crossed the Russian frontier at Lublin, Szmuness decided to return to Poland. Compatriots at the Polish Embassy urged him to return, arguing that it was his duty, since Hitler had killed so many people that there were only a few people with professional qualifications left in Poland. As a doctor he would be guaranteed a good position and a good apartment. So, on May 25, 1959, Wolf Szmuness returned to his native land, with entrance permit number 087806. It was not the happiest of homecomings. Despite the promises there was no job, no apartment, and, most terrible of all, no family. All his relatives had perished in the Warsaw ghetto and nothing remained from his past. Living in one room, in a building without any windows, he and his wife found life so hard that they were ready to return. But they knew it would be Siberia again, really the end of the road. Finally Szmuness found a job in Lublin, where he continued his work in public health, epidemiology, and, most important, hepatitis.

He kept abreast of scientific and medical developments by reading whatever Western literature he could obtain. He corresponded with Dr. Robert McCollum of Yale University, a distinguished scientist in hepatitis B, and so learned of the pioneer studies by Baruch Blumberg, Fred Prince, and Saul Krugman leading to a test that revealed the virus in the blood. When Szmuness, in the 1960s, learned that the hepatitis B virus had been described in structure and functional complexity, he knew that it would be only a matter of time before a vaccine would be discovered, though he could not have predicted how awkward the virus would prove to be. Immediately he began a series of seminal studies to reveal the patterns of hepatitis B infection in populations because he well knew that it is not enough to cure just one individual. Success in medicine comes only when whole populations are cured or, better still, protected. It is at this interface between the individual and the population that the skills and understanding of an epidemiologist are crucial and it was Szmuness's studies of the disease patterns that made him supremely qualified for the job that the future would hold.

Slowly life improved and by most standards the family lived well. Though anti-Semitism was rife, Szmuness was to discover that there were other, happier attitudes around. One summer he took a ten-day holiday at a state resort in the mountains, where he shared a room with another man. They got on famously, taking long walks over the mountains, eating their meals together, always arguing and discussing. At the end of the time, his new friend said: "Since we are leaving tomorrow, I have something I must tell you, for I have not been entirely open. You must know that I am a Catholic and actually, I am about to become a bishop.

But I felt that this knowledge might have been embarrassing for you as a Jew, and I didn't want anything to disturb our happy days together."

Szmuness laughed, insisting that this knowledge wouldn't have affected him at all. They corresponded for a year or so and although he never forgot that "wise and radiant man," he wasn't to see him for many years, not, in fact, until the cardinal chamberlain at the Vatican, came onto the balcony to announce the name of the new pope. As he watched television, Szmuness suddenly grabbed his wife. "I know that man . . . my friend . . . in the mountains."*

Although opportunities for research were limited and chances of advancement practically nil, Szmuness did make progress in his career. His first major success came in 1967, when an epidemic of enteric fever, that claimed thousands of victims, struck a small town in the Tatry mountains on the Czechoslovakian border. Called in to investigate, he quickly discovered that the central water supply had been contaminated with sewage. Suddenly he was a celebrity and the Polish newspapers praised him to the skies. Within the year the very same papers were calling him a traitor.

In 1967 the Six-Day War broke out between Egypt and Israel and anti-Semitic feelings overflowed in Poland. Szmuness was ordered to attend a rally and publicly add his protests against Israel. He said he would not. Given until 6:00 P.M. that day to change his mind, he refused once more. The next morning, when he arrived at his offices first at the university and then at the Public Health Institute, letters of dismissal were waiting on both desks and instantly he was a nonperson.

Maya Szmuness had anticipated this and had already begun planning. That evening she heard the heavy step in the corridor and her husband entered, dead white. "Maya," he said heavily, "I have lost my jobs." "Okay," she replied briskly, "now I'm the head of the family. First you will take a rest and then we will go to Israel or America."

They withdrew to a small village some way from Lublin and waited for official approval to leave the country. Since the Szmunesses had been saving for six years to buy a car, they had some ready money, but since they had to live and bribe officials, and arrange to sell their property, it was quickly gone. Finally, they received visas and were given one month

* Pope John Paul, the former Karol Wojtyla, never forgot Szmuness either. Years later, Helena Szmuness, then a newspaper correspondent, was covering Cardinal Wojtyla's visit to New York. On hearing her name the Cardinal asked her if her father was a scientist. When she said yes, he replied, "Then we spent ten days together in the mountains, many years ago. He is a marvelous man. Give him my greetings."

to get out. From Lublin they went to Vienna, from Vienna to Rome where, under the auspices of the Hebrew Immigrant Aid Society, they applied to the U.S. Embassy for visas. Finally, on a bitter, snowy day in February 1969, they landed at Kennedy Airport, with only $15 in their pockets, having lost everything – country, home, job, and dignity.

The next day Maya Szmuness found a job in a factory and for six months sewed neckties. She now loathes ties. Wolf Szmuness knocked on doors and wrote letters to medical agencies, to the few doctors he had corresponded with, and to others he did not even know, such as Walsh McDermott. He walked the streets, scanned the want ads, read in the medical libraries, and became more and more depressed. On the roller coaster of their lives, he was at the bottom once again. Approaching fifty, it seemed hopeless to try to reconstruct his scientific career, so he was on the verge of taking a job in a pocketbook factory.

Then one day in late spring 1969, he was reading in the library of Cornell University Medical College when an announcement boomed through the public address system: "If Dr. Wolf Szmuness is here, will he please go to Dr. Walsh McDermott's office." Of all the people to whom he had written, it was the sensitive, compassionate Walsh McDermott who had acted.

That evening Maya returned from work to Room 629 in the cheap, tatty hotel on Broadway to find an ecstatic Wolf. "I saw so much food on the table and Wolf say: 'Maya, we have Passover. I got a job.' I said, 'What kind of job?' He said, 'I don't know. But I be working in Blood Center. It's good enough. I know I make it.' So I say, 'How much the salary?' and Wolf say: 'I don't know. I forgot to ask!' We were dancing in that room."

He began work on April 29, and a few days later Aaron Kellner saw him in the corridor.

Szmuness would always regard the sequence of events that led him to the New York Blood Center as miraculous, and those of the next few years were equally so. In a very real sense he was "home" for the first time in his entire life. To begin with, he was lucky that fate had placed him in this particular research institution, of the multitude of research centers in the United States. Most are big, impersonal, bureaucratic, and competitive – sometimes aggressively so. But the New York Blood Center has the warm ambience of a small family whose individual members might at times disagree, even bitterly, but where the atmosphere remains friendly, loyal, and supportive. The characteristics of any scientific institution are mostly determined by its leadership. In Dr. Aaron Kellner the Blood Center has a director of benign toughness, good business acumen, a deeply compassionate clinician who understands the importance of basic research and who sees his job as twofold. His first goal is to run the day-to-day affairs of the Blood Center efficiently and prudently so that its service to the wider New York community can be maintained. His second aim is not to tell his scientists what to do but to find out what *they* want to do, and then ensure that they have the means. Blood is the Blood Center's business – they extract, purify, donate, sell, investigate, separate, and discuss it, then write scientific papers – and now the Center is recognized as one of the most distinguished scientific institutions in the world.

Here Szmuness thrived, like many others before and since. Here he met as colleagues many pioneers in hepatitis. Fred Prince was one. Saul Krugman, by then approaching seventy, was another, a gentle man with whom Szmuness established an immediate loving rapport. With Bob McCollum he had already had a transatlantic correspondence of eight years' duration, started by a letter from McCollum who had read one of Szmuness's publications. McCollum recalls that the correspondence suddenly ceased and the man seemed to disappear from the scene, until one day in late 1969, at a conference in New York, a gnomelike figure, with a shock of yellow hair and a craggy, lined face, touched him on the arm, grinned, and said, "Hello, I'm Wolf Szmuness."

These brilliant people with whom Szmuness now associated were in for some surprises. "Within a very short time," Aaron Kellner recalls,

Dr. Prince realized that we had a most unusual man in our midst, one with extraordinary insights and capabilities. So he gave him progressively more and more freedom and responsibility. Soon Wolf was designing his own projects, then given his own lab, and within five years – in 1974 – we created a separate Department of Epidemiology which he headed. Similarly, he was first appointed a lecturer at the School of Public Health of Columbia, and in what must be record time he was leap-frogged to full professor.

Next he collected his own staff around him: Cladd Stevens, a young pediatrician, had been studying the patterns of hepatitis B infection among mothers and children in Taiwan, and joined Wolf as second-in-command; on the nonscientific side Ed Harley and Allison Brennan were to play central roles in his important studies. "I was an actress and a writer," Allison Brennan says, "and of course these two lucrative trades meant that I had to do a little supplementing. So I showed up as a tem-

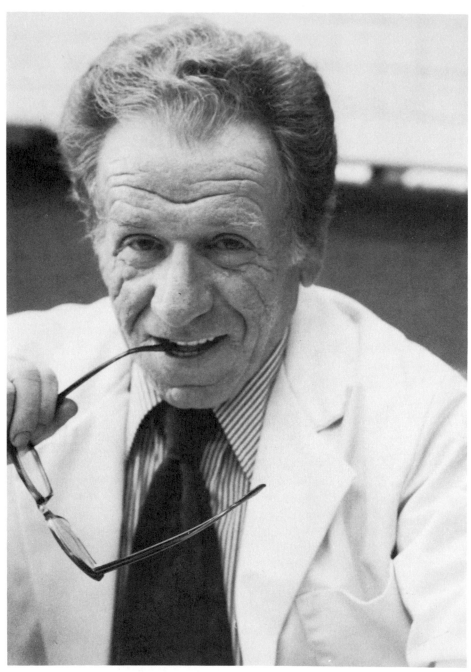

Dr. Wolf Szmuness. (Donna Harley)

porary typist and helped Dr. Szmuness with his first papers. They were so full of terrible grammatical problems that I insisted on rewriting them and so he hired me to work for him."

Szmuness now began to expand in all directions – physically, scientifically, and spiritually. He would often talk, with incredulity, of the freedom to speak his mind without fear and to move about at will. He relished the joys of living in the United States and plunged into the experiences it had to offer. He acquired his first car, then his first house, then his first sailboat, all enjoyed with a childlike jubilation. He grew in emotional stature and personal command. He savored fresh experiences. For a while he dressed in mod fashion and, for an even briefer period, took up jogging, much to the amusement of all his friends. Then much to their relief, he quit. As his confidence grew, so did his dry, teasing, deadpan humor, but so too did his stubbornness and his brief flashes of anger. For so much important work had to be done, with so much time to make up, that he would not tolerate anything that fell short of his towering standards of perfection and meticulousness. Years before Maya had learned how to bide her time and manœuver her way, and soon, so too did Cladd Stevens and his other colleagues and staff. As for Aaron Kellner and Saul Krugman, Szmuness came to hold them in deep affection and they, in their turn, came to love and cherish the small craggy man who had suddenly appeared in their lives.

With a series of brilliant papers on hepatitis infections, Szmuness's career progressed by leaps and bounds. Soon he had an international reputation. He was phenomenally successful by any standards, including (Kellner remarks) the great American litmus test for measuring scientific success: the ability to command grant support. But he could never believe his own success and was never secure in his confidence. It was as if he still feared that this newfound happiness would suddenly be snatched away. This uncertainty revealed itself frequently. He regularly complained to Kellner that his laboratory was skirting the brink of insolvency while Kellner, on the other hand, had the impression that people were lined up outside his door waving checks, pleading with him to undertake projects. "And," says Kellner, "that was pretty close to the truth. Wolf eventually had the largest staff and by far the largest budget of any research lab at the Blood Center."

He would never completely exorcise his past. Its ghosts still haunted his sleep and on one occasion the memories overpowered him. His early years at the Blood Center marked the period of détente when annual scientific exchanges were planned between the Soviet Union and the United States. After two exploratory meetings, it became clear that hepatitis was an excellent area where cooperative programs would be fruitful. If the Americans were to discuss hepatitis with the Russians, then clearly one man who had to be present was Wolf Szmuness. So in 1975 Kellner invited him to join the U.S. delegation and present a paper in Moscow.

Kellner had problems on two fronts simultaneously: the Soviets wouldn't give Szmuness a visa and Szmuness didn't want one. The Soviets were told: no Szmuness, no conference. Then Kellner turned to tackle his friend.

He adamantly refused. Nothing was going to get him to the Soviet Union. He was absolutely certain that once there he would never get out again. I tried in a hundred different ways to convince him that as an American citizen the State Department would protect him, but he wouldn't budge. So other members of the delegation joined in and reluctantly and grudgingly he finally agreed to go. As the departure date approached, Wolf became increasingly anxious and agitated. He complained of splitting headaches, stomach distress, heart palpitations, diarrhea, skin rashes – the whole spectrum of psychosomatic disorders. Eventually we got him to the airplane – very apprehensive, very reluctant – and the trip was entirely uneventful. We arrived at Chermetiego airport in Moscow, debarked, and walked into the terminal building. Wolf and I brought up the rear. As we opened the door there was a tall Red Army soldier. It was the beginning of winter and he had on a long coat almost down to his ankles, a gun in his arms, and he was standing rigidly at attention. Wolf took one look, his knees turned to water and he collapsed – flat on the ground. We revived him in a few minutes and he was all for going straight back. But we convinced him that the State Department had assured us there was no way the Russians could keep him, and eventually he began, slowly, to believe us, got to his feet and we went through Customs.

There was a fairly stereotyped ritual on these trips. On the day after arrival each side presented a series of papers but we were usually talking at each other rather than with each other so discussion was generally quite perfunctory. Wolf's paper was scheduled for the afternoon. The morning presentations were given before an audience of no more than forty people in a hall that held three hundred, but when we returned after lunch we were surprised to find the auditorium jammed. The big guns in hepatitis in the Soviet Union had turned out en masse and they were heavily loaded. Szmuness, speaking in Russian, gave one of his usually brilliant presentations, beautifully organized and solidly documented. When the discussion was open there was a parade of speakers, each giving unsolicited papers of five to fifteen minutes in length, aimed at refuting his findings and denigrating the work. Wolf listened quietly, occasionally shaking his head and taking a few notes, while we squirmed uncomfortably. When the barrage had spent itself the chairman invited Wolf to respond. He rose slowly, put his head

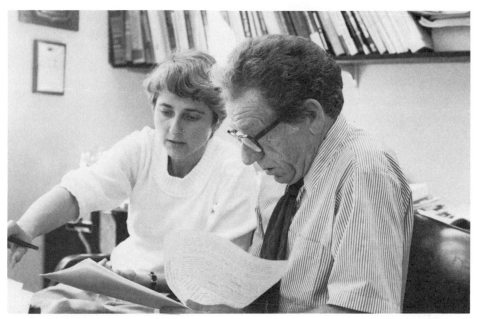

Dr. Wolf Szmuness and Dr. Cladd Stevens discussing the trial data. (Donna Harley)

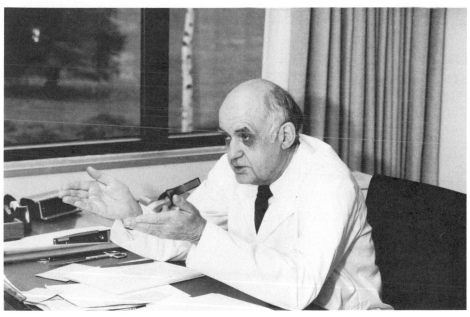

Dr. Maurice R. Hilleman, Director of the Merck Institute for Therapeutic Research, explains the development of the hepatitis B vaccine.
(Merck Institute for Therapeutic Research)

down as he usually did and instead of going to the rostrum, stayed on the floor directly in front of the audience. He first turned to us, his colleagues, in the front row and apologized for speaking in Russian: he would fill us in later. He then calmly proceeded with his point-by-point rebuttal. I should add that to be rebutted by Wolf Szmuness was like being run over by a Sherman tank. He never stooped to *ad hominem* argument, but the precision of his logic and his ability to marshal facts were overwhelming and often devastating. As he warmed to his task, pacing slowly up and back on the floor, we knew, without understanding a word, that the Russians were being cannonaded. As he built to a climax I was reminded of Tchaikovsky's 1812 Overture and its relentless crescendo. When he finished, he politely thanked the audience for their interest, and sat down. There was a moment's hushed silence, and then the Russians rose as a man and gave Wolf a standing ovation.

Others beside Szmuness were to regard his joining the Blood Center as miraculous. For he was to design and execute what has been described as the finest clinical field trial in the history of medicine, one that tested a vaccine for hepatitis B. His timing was impeccable because the five years between his arrival and his becoming head of the Laboratory of Epidemiology in 1974 were the years when the dream came true and a hepatitis B vaccine was developed. Certainly Szmuness had anticipated this possibility years before, but meanwhile virologists had been through an extremely frustrating period. The organisms that cause most childhood diseases, such as polio and diphtheria, can be cultured in the laboratory and so vaccines prepared relatively easily. But other viruses are horribly refractory, and hepatitis B is one.

The scientists tried another tack. The traces of viral protein, those flecks from the overcoat of the virus (the Dane particles, so named after the English doctor who first described them) are present in great quantity in the blood of carriers, and it is these that provoke a protective immune response. Dr. Baruch Blumberg and his colleague, Dr. Miller, suggested that if these flecks could be extracted from the blood of carriers, then concentrated, purified, and sterilized, they might be used as a vaccine.

Dr. Saul Krugman and his colleagues at the New York University Medical Center followed up this suggestion, extracting the protein, diluting it with water, and inactivating it by heating. In 1973 they gave this vaccine to mentally retarded children about to be institutionalized at the Willowbrook Hospital, Staten Island, New York City, a closed community where over and over again cycles of epidemics smouldered and raged. After being vaccinated with this extract, 70 percent of the children were totally protected from attacks of hepatitis B. Thus it was shown that even after the hepatitis B virus was killed, its protein could *still* be recognized by the immune system and protective antibodies made. An effective vaccine *was* possible, but it would be a unique and unusual one, for the patients who had the disease would be the source of protection for those who might get it.

Under the direction of Maurice B. Hilleman, at the Merck Institute for Therapeutic Research, at West Point, Pennsylvania, the scientific teams went to work. The commercial vaccine that they produced eventually cost, by some estimates, as much as $70 million to develop, over a period of fourteen years. Going through seven separate stages, from extraction to animal testing, it once took sixty-five weeks to make a commercial batch. The first step was to extract the serum from the blood of volunteer gay men, who were carriers of the disease.

The process used, *plasmaphoresis*, a procedure by which blood plasma is extracted and the viral particles recovered, is complicated and potentially very dangerous. Handling the infectious serum is risky for one twentieth-billionth part of one liter could infect a roomful of people. So from the moment the needle is inserted into the vein of a volunteer until the moment of injection, possibly months later, when another needle slides into a sealed phial of vaccine, *everything* is done in an entirely closed system. Human hands cannot touch the stuff, and the most stringent safety precautions ensure that as many barriers as possible are maintained between the serum and the outside world.

There is no way to extract a person's blood serum without taking the red blood cells too. These the scientists don't want and the volunteers are glad to have back. So before a volunteer is connected to the needle, he signs his name on the sealed bag that will receive his blood. Once full, this is spun so fast in the centrifuge that the red blood cells separate out. The faintly yellow serum on top is siphoned off and the bag, now containing red blood cells only, is taken back to the volunteer who confirms his signature. The cells are returned into his vein in a solution of normal saline and then another batch of blood is taken from him, and the whole process repeated.

The volunteer is now free to leave, but the months of work on his serum now begins. It is decanted into another bag that is sealed, wrapped, folded, and placed into an ordinary can. This lid is annealed into place just as if the scientists were canning tomatoes, and a label bearing the name and date is stuck on. All the cans taken on any one day are now carefully packed into cardboard boxes, which are sealed in their turn. A truck picks up the boxes and under close guard drives away from the Blood

Center, over to the west side of Manhattan Island, under the Hudson River and down the New Jersey turnpike to West Point, Pennsylvania.

Once there the cans enter a biohazard area, a facility where workers must be gowned and masked and wear sterile gloves. The cans are now opened automatically, by remote control, and all labels, whether on them or the wrapping boxes, are destroyed so no one knows from which individual the sample came. There are fourteen similar donor centers across the United States, and the sera from all volunteers are put into churns where the process of extracting the critical particles now begins.

The industrial process to make the vaccine consists of four separate operations that first isolate the essential particles, then purify, concentrate, and finally – and most critically – inactivate them. Once made, though, the vaccine has to be tested for purity. Next it is tested for potency, to ensure that it provokes only an immune response but not an infection. Chimpanzees are used for these tests, since they are the only animals that contract human hepatitis B. Two animal colonies were used by the New York Blood Center, one in Louisiana and another on an island off the coast of Liberia. The animals don't die, either from the vaccine test or from hepatitis B, but, once tested, they are not killed. The Louisiana colony lives out its normal lifespan in a chimpanzees' "senior citizens home" and the Liberian animals are gradually readapted to the wild. This process of readaptation is very difficult. It takes years, much longer than it takes to make the vaccine, and in both cases the costs to the drug company are very high.

Such procedures show that the vaccine is safe and that no other living organisms are present. But, as Dr. Maurice Hilleman (Director, Merck Institute for Therapeutic Research) points out, no vaccine can be proved totally safe in a laboratory: it has to be shown to be so in human subjects. Thus testing in human beings followed next, and with great perspicacity Merck provided volunteers for the first human safety trials from among its executives and staff. Then further safety and immunologic studies began, involving several hundred human volunteers. The focus had to shift from experimental animals and individual volunteers to human populations. To answer the simple but fundamental question – Does this vaccine protect large populations against the disease? – calls for a clinical trial in a human population, designed so carefully that there is no ambiguity whatever about the answer. It must be a clear-cut "yes" or "no."

It is in the skill with which an epidemiologist eliminates ambiguity in a clinical trial that brilliance is demonstrated and success measured. But eliminating ambiguity is not as easy as it might appear, and it was here that his colleagues at the Blood Center consider it miraculous that Szmuness was at hand. In 1982 Aaron Kellner told me why:

What Wolf brings to science is a mind that works like a steel trap – a mind that is clear, that asks direct, proper questions and that is capable of finding answers for those questions in an unambiguous fashion. When he got through with an experiment or writing a paper or presenting an argument there were no more questions to be asked. He also brings an impeccable tough-minded honesty and doesn't fool himself. His experiments either demonstrate what they're supposed to or they are discarded and new ones are designed. Many other people were doing epidemiological studies in hepatitis. None of them was as complete, none as solid, none as thoroughly convincing as Szmuness's.

Szmuness himself had the clearest of visions, knowing both what preliminary epidemiologic studies had to be done before the trial could even begin and how to design it so that the greatest amount of information would then be elicited. But one might wonder why any preliminary studies were necessary. Why not just divide a population at random, give half the vaccine and half a placebo, and at the end of several months see who had become ill with hepatitis B? Szmuness wanted more definitive results, ones absolutely clear-cut; he needed to find a group in which the odds of getting such results were greater than in any other. Preliminary studies would direct him to an "ideal" population for the trial, one that met a number of accepted criteria. It is rare for any population to meet them all, however.

First, since the results of a clinical trial are always expressed statistically, an ideal population is one large enough to give a valid result: a thousand people are better than ten. Next, the ideal population has a high attack rate of the disease: one where 1 person in 3 in the group is likely to catch the infection is better than if only 1 in 100 people do. Third, the ideal group is easily identifiable and reasonably homogeneous: it is not dispersed throughout the whole of society and does not consist of, say, young *and* old, male *and* female, sick *and* ill, celibate *and* promiscuous, static *and* mobile all mixed up. Fourth, such a population is both young *and* healthy so that other diseases won't interfere with the clinical data to be elicited. Finally, the ideal group is accessible, so follow-up tests that may spread over two years can be easily carried out. These were the characteristics that Wolf Szmuness sought.

Between 1973 and 1978 Szmuness ran a series of crucial baseline studies, both within and outside the United States. He found out who was mostly at risk from hepatitis B, where the major pools of infection were, how many carriers existed, whether the amount of sexual activity affected the incidence of the disease. Most important, he found his ideal group for a clinical trial. Sexually active, urban gay men met *all* the criteria: they had a rate of hepatitis B infection nearly ten times that in the general population of the country; they were a compact, homogeneous group and stood out clearly; they existed on his doorstep; they were young and presumably healthy; through their institutions – churches, synagogues, professional associations, health forums and clubs – they were accessible; they didn't tend to move around and there were a large number of them in a compact area just across town, in Greeenwich Village on the west side of New York.

Szmuness was now poised for his finest hour. All the elements for success were present – a vaccine, impeccable baseline studies, an intelligent and highly motivated trial population, a professional staff, and wonderful moral and financial support. Recognizing that fortune had determined that he would be the right man in the right place at the right time, Szmuness seized his opportunity with both hands and, in 1978, began detailed planning for a double blind trial of the hepatitis B vaccine.

His trial population, whose members would remain strictly anonymous, would be randomly divided: one half would receive the vaccine, the other a useless placebo, and the differences in the disease patterns of the two measured. It sounds easy but actually Szmuness had to execute a plan of formidable logistic dimensions involving thousands of people. He had to work out his strategy in the finest detail with regard to the numbers and sequence of injections, the dosages, the follow-up blood tests, the analyses and recordkeeping, for he had to elicit as much information as possible. Once the strategy was determined then, ideally, the trial would be executed without any deviations. Failure to do a follow-up test at a specific time might throw doubt upon the validity of the final result.

Behind all his planning lay three important principles that are built into all field trials: (1) their events must be totally controlled; (2) the vaccine and placebo groups must be assigned absolutely anonymously and at random; and (3) the trial has to be double blind so it can be obvious that no biases have entered, either into the selection of patients or the interpretation of the results. "Double blind" meant that not even the volunteers or the staffs, or the doctors, not even Wolf Szmuness himself, would know who was getting the vaccine and who the placebo. Secrecy would be set up by means of a code; volunteers would be identified by numbers, not names; and only two people, the officers responsible for the safety of the trial, would have the knowledge to break the code.

Szmuness had his ideal group all right, but not all its members would qualify as suitable for the trial. He needed at least eight hundred people and preferably one thousand, but they must never have had hepatitis B in the past, or be carriers, or have active disease now. Since gay men are constantly exposed to hepatitis B, he would have to screen thousands in order to find the suitable one thousand. He and his staff were in for months of sustained effort in which perverse, creative, emotional human beings would be asked or cajoled into doing certain things at certain times, without exception or deviation.

Other, quite different, imperatives came to bear. All clinical trials become enmeshed with social considerations, but in this case they would be of a very special and difficult kind, considerations arising from the need to deal with a socially unacceptable group who felt alienated. Subjecting these people to sensitive questions of great intimacy about their sex life would present difficulties of a kind not usually encountered; getting co-operation from men who had every reason for secrecy and withdrawal would be very difficult, for many still led secret lives. They practiced their professions during working hours, whether as bankers, doctors, priests, policemen, writers, actors, restaurateurs, or bureaucrats, but in the evenings would retreat to the haunts of the Village and the Christopher Street Pier, areas where they lived another life under a veil of anonymity they might be desperate to preserve.

As well as fear, he might face cynicism from them, gay men being under no illusions that the surge of interest in hepatitis B reflected a genuine concern for *their* health problems. But hepatitis B was a disease of the medical community too, and the blood of 25 percent of all practicing physicians had evidence of prior exposure. The virus all too easily passes through those institutions where blood is used, whether general hospitals or special divisions such as dialysis units. Patients on immunotherapy, cancer patients, and hemophiliacs were all at risk, as well as the poorer people in society. But none of these groups were as easily accessible as gay men, nor did any of them meet the criteria for the ideal population so completely. There was no alternative: Szmuness had to get to know and understand gay men.

Nothing in Wolf Szmuness's background or experience had prepared him for the encounters that were to follow. Shy, extraordinarily naïve, and in certain respects innocent, he was ignorant of all aspects of gay culture. Though he certainly knew the meaning of the word "homosexual," there his knowledge ended and he would, in turn, be baffled, bewildered, and sometimes distressed by what he was to learn.

He had little idea of what was involved, and it was Allison Brennan who undertook to enlighten him. She remembers:

Shortly after I showed up, I typed that paper of Wolf's on the sexual transmission of disease that showed us how dire their situation was. The months passed and I participated in some of the studies and the time came when he wanted to start the vaccine trial. Suddenly he needed several thousand blood samples from a community that up to this point had experienced massive discrimination. It was pretty clear to me that he was approaching this problem in his usual delightful, naïve way.

So one day I said to him: "You know, Dr. Szmuness, this is not a blood donor population that is just going to give you a teaspoon of blood for some strange research. This is a vast community and you are going to want thousands upon thousands of blood samples. You are not going to be able to do it in the normal way. You are going to have to launch a PR campaign; you are going to have to involve the gay community; you are going to have to get the movement to be a part of this whole program."

He looked at me straight as he usually did, without comment – you couldn't quite tell what he thought. Then a few days later said, "Very vell, Allison, you vill do it."

So Allison did it. It just happened that being an actress and being a writer gave me experiences that really fitted and certainly I knew a lot about hepatitis by then. Finally I was in charge of getting thousands of men into the study and educating everybody about what hepatitis was, what our problems were, and making certain everyone was happy. They gave me the title of Director of Recruitment, Education and Community Relations, simply to give me clout when I went about my business.

Initially we worked with the Gay Men's Health Project and got volunteers to give that extra teaspoonful of blood. But by the spring of 1978, when we began the massive screening to find the 850 suitable men we mounted a massive PR campaign and started with the Bloodmobiles. These are enormous vans which travel all round the city, going to the blood donors rather than have them come to the Blood Center. But now we took the Bloodmobiles all over the place – to the gay bars, down to the pier on the West Side where the gay men congregate, and caught a lot of people who were just going to sunbathe. We would haul them into the Bloodmobile and invite them to take a blood test.

[Asked whether mobile vampires was their image, Brennan continues:] "Exactly. As a matter of fact we had a picture of Dracula in the Bloodmobile to inspire people and make them feel comfortable, and one of the volunteers had a set of vampire teeth that he brought along too. If a guy agreed to take part in the initial screening program we gave him an ID number, and an ID card, and told him *never* to lose it. For from then on he would be known to us only by that number. We had to ask the guys lots of intimate questions too, not only about how old they were and what illnesses they'd had or were having, but when did their active gay life begin and how many sexual contacts they'd had over the past year. These could run between 200 and 700 a year – the average was about 360.

The men, equally, had so many questions for the staff that they were given a brochure titled, "What You Should Know about Hepatitis B in Gay Men, and the New York Hepatitis B Vaccine." Written by Dr. Cladd Stevens, it explained why hepatitis was a common problem and why its incidence increased in men with a significantly large number of sexual partners (the group they needed for the trial), and why the trial had to be double blind, and how the participants would be protected if there were complications. After the blood had been taken and the ID number registered, a man was told to return in a week for the results. Then, if the test had shown no active or previous hepatitis, he would be asked to sign up.

The initial burden of the recruitment drive fell on a gay man, Mitchell Speer, and then on the new project manager of the Blood Center's trial program, John Morrison. Other staff included Mike Kieran, a male nurse, Liz de Kosto, Jane Brown, Marji McQueen, Arthur Brown, and twenty more volunteers. They sought the men everywhere: in the streets, churches, at the meetings of activist groups. They blanketed the gay community with photographs, posters, leaflets, displays, advertisements; they covered the annual Gay Parade; they asked the rabbis to speak in the synagogues. So, as the year passed, recruits began to sign up in a whole variety of places, from the Christopher Street pier to headquarters organizations like Identity House, the Gay Youth of New York, and various religious groups. Yet the Bloodmobile and the Gay Men's Health Project were the places where most people would enroll.

Mitchell Speer remembers the task as a challenge of a kind he had never had before. He'd been appointed early on, so found himself one of a small team that needed to recruit a large number of people. By the time John Morrison joined Speer was exhausted and weighted down under the burden of decision. But the chemistry between the two men was incredible and from then on, things began to move rapidly. Speer is hyperactive; Morrison calm. Speer is impulsive and would want to get in touch with Szmuness immediately if something was not working; Morrison would relax and wait. Speer is a nervous perfectionist; Morrison a calm and efficient realist. And Morrison became the prime liaison between the Gay Men's Health Project and the New York Blood Center.

Szmuness, too, made his own contacts. He invited all the community leaders – the clergy from the gay churches, the owners of the bathhouses, the writers attached to gay publications – to a gathering at the Blood Center to discuss the disease and to tell them about the prospects for protection and to gauge what cooperation he might expect. Cheese and wine were served at the reception. Though Szmuness alone spoke, his deputy, Cladd Stevens was nervous. As she recalls,

I had never met a gay man before to the best of my knowledge. I was worried about our reception, about how I would behave, even that we might embarrass them. I didn't even know how to look a gay man in the eye. But it was remarkably relaxed and everyone was totally adjusted, even when Wolf slipped up while describing some initial data and referred to the difference between "gay" and "normal" populations. But this just got a big laugh.

She believes that there were two reasons for the cooperation the gay community quickly extended: they recognized the full extent of their problem, that it was an epidemic disease with no treatment, and were anxious to gain a better social image. But everyone knew they were walking a tightrope. Too much publicity about the trial could lead to accusations that gay men spread hepatitis everywhere; on the other hand, if things went well, the community could certainly use some credit.

It was Dr. Dan William, one of the founding members of the Gay Men's Health Project, who first used the term "symbiotic relationship" to describe what now developed. Like many other gay men he was late in acknowledging his sexual proclivities and after finishing medical school chose an internship in New York City, he says, "primarily to fill the need I had to be honest to myself and to other people." He was to play a major role in the trial, being not only the physician appointed to care for the gay men, but a member of the Advisory Board as well. His scientific experience and his perceptive understanding of his own social group told him that the time was ripe now for the trial. "It couldn't have happened a decade before," he says, "because there was no gay community, no gay health facilities, no identifiable gay leaders who could draw gay people together. We had something the Blood Center wanted – a motivated, intelligent, cohesive group – and they had something we very much wanted – a way of controlling this disease. We both fulfilled each other's needs in a manner that was constructive and beneficial."

If Szmuness's scientific brilliance lay in identifying this community in the first place, his personal humanity showed itself in one attitude that he consistently made plain to all: anyone who participates in a clinical field trial deserves the highest consideration and respect. Although he never came to understand why someone became a homosexual, his sensitivity was shown in hundreds of ways. He appointed mostly gay men to his staff. Dr. Dan William was on the advisory board. Two gay physicians were coinvestigators in all the research, their names appeared on the published papers, and all changes in protocols were discussed with them first. He showed concern in practical ways too. Because the only income came from donations, the Gay Men's Health Project was housed in a seedy building where the rent was low. They had one room, consisting of a series of makeshift areas separated by curtains, with wooden benches and a wooden floor. Szmuness gave money for couches, cushions, an orange carpet, for Japanese lanterns to hang from the ceiling, and wooden cubicles for private medical examinations.

To deepen his understanding of the people whose cooperation was so vital, Szmuness wanted to know about their personalities and their lives, so he was taken to their homes and haunts, baths, and brothels. The whole range from love to perversion was shown to him, a range no different in character and extent than for heterosexuals. A cynic might argue that his concern was a facade, a device used to capture a group of people he badly needed, but none of the gay men think so. They both admired him for his professional skills and were grateful for his personal concerns.

Thus for two or three years Szmuness and his staff moved between two worlds. Across the main theme of the clinical trial they would be responding to two starkly contrasting counterpoints. The world of the Blood Center was calm – totally undramatic actually, Stevens insists. Clean, aseptic, fresh, and ordered, its scientific and medical routines were woven into a life that had the quality of a quiet, melodic string quartet.

But then they would cross town and plunge into the syncopated, jazzy, frenetic world of Christopher Street's dirty sidewalks, a world whose harsh rhythms were at one and the same time vibrant and stale, exhilarating and tatty. The dissonances of the unique mixture of people and nationalities, occupations and outlooks sometimes grated. For Allison Brennan, who lived in Greenwich Village, it was familiar country, but for Wolf Szmuness and Cladd Stevens this was a very strange land and *they* were the foreigners.

Spring 1978 moved into summer and the annual Gay Day Parade rolled down the streets. Fall yielded to Christmas and jingle bells, and still enrollment continued. Two kinds of problems now surfaced – some faced the volunteers, others the recruiters – and one could not be alleviated at all. Before a preliminary screening no one mentioned that if hepatitis B *was* found this could mean a man was a carrier, with a potential to infect others forever. No man could be told his state at the time of his first test

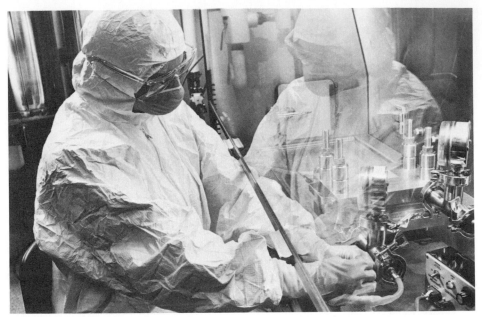

The commercial process of vaccine production must take place under the most rigorous conditions of containment.
(Merck Institute for Therapeutic Research)

because there is no way to know immediately: the virus must remain in the blood for at least six months for the carrier state to be confirmed. But this created a major crisis and one man became wildly angry. Had he known the test would reveal the carrier state he wouldn't have taken it. Indeed he didn't want to know, because knowing meant his life was now irrevocably changed and he felt he could no more have sex than if he had syphilis or gonorrhea. The vaccine wouldn't help him either since, like most vaccines, it was expected only to prevent infection, not treat the disease.

Then, despite the anonymous ID numbers, other volunteers became reluctant to have their names on forms, computer runs, and printouts. "The gay community has a healthy paranoia about purges," John Morrison explained. "They were unwilling to do anything *now* which would enable them to be identified later if, for example, a combination of groups like the Moral Majority and the John Birch Society gained political control in the United States." Confidentiality thus became even more critical and was well covered. Szmuness and Stevens were scrupulous in the way letters were sent out: no names were ever revealed. The members of the two Review Committees on Safety and General Advice saw only the computer runs and statistics: the gay recruiters alone knew the names of the gay men they signed up.

Safety was a third concern, being guinea pigs a fourth. Of course, everyone knew that the vaccine had been tested in chimpanzees and in more than two hundred human volunteers. Moreover, they were also shown that the particular vaccine to be used, *Merck Hepatitis B vaccine, Lot No. 751*, had been given to a further twenty-eight people in the Merck company and in a close follow-up that lasted over six months, no one complained of anything more than a sore arm. But still the volunteers worried, for being made from the blood of carriers, the vaccine *was* completely unlike any other. So might it not provoke hepatitis B, or might they not catch other infectious diseases from these human factories? The fact that many Merck employees had volunteered to receive the vaccine remained the single most comforting evidence. It allayed fears, for if there was any question of danger, these Merck volunteers would undoubtedly have been the first to raise the issue.

Medical care was a final worry. Who would pay for the treatment of men contracting hepatitis B during the trial, and would those who developed other forms of hepatitis be taken care of as well? Szmuness promised that anyone who acquired any hepatitis would receive free medical care from Dan William — and they did. This, too, was a wise decision:

gay people in the trial were happy to be cared for by a gay physician. And the Blood Center doctors were pleased because in William they had a clinical observer who would not only see all cases as they developed, but one who could monitor the symptoms through a sustained period. So for the very first time in history doctors obtained a detailed and prolonged look at the course of hepatitis B. Most doctors who see the disease have a skewed picture, since patients present themselves late, when they are already sick with symptoms. Dan William was to see people who, though at first asymptomatic, had blood enzymes that showed the virus was present. He followed them, as they became sick and got better or as they became carriers. Since biologic samples were taken constantly, a clinical and physiologic profile of the disease has been drawn from beginning to end and will be of inestimable value in the future, especially since all extremes of the disease turned up, from the mildest form to the most severe.

The recruiters' concerns boiled down to one hard fact: sufficient volunteers simply weren't coming in. Further massive recruitment was necessary and the next push was more sensitively designed, with the community overwhelmingly covered. The thrust of the recruitment campaign was changed. Allison Brennan describes the change:

We had started with very responsible political gay organizations and handed out very serious literature. We had placed advertisements in every kind of gay newspaper or magazine that you can imagine. We had public service announcements and we designed all kinds of serious flyers and posters and blitzed these all over the town.

But once we had covered the several hundred serious, responsible people, we then moved into everybody's sex life. So we created the next pamphlet with a lively headline "Is Variety the Spice of Your Sex Life?" This implied that if you want to keep up sex and not worry, you had better get this test for hepatitis B, because there's nothing gay about being sick. And since an ounce of prevention is better than anything else, why not do yourself a favor and be screened for possible participation in the trial?

Then we really hit the streets. We hit the bars and we hit the baths, and we hit hard. We went to "Man's Country" and other similar bathhouses and took blood samples right in there. This was utterly wild because sometimes the men appeared with their towels on and sometimes not. Liz and I were both there and Mike Kieran, the nurse, and the guys would come out of whatever room they had just been in and line up to have their blood samples taken and answer all the unbelievable questions we had to ask.

One time we were taken upstairs to a nicely carpeted suite on the same floor as one of their "fantasy rooms." I know it had a fire engine in it but I don't know what else because I didn't look. But there was one guy who turned on in the fantasy room, and somehow wandered down the hall. He took one glazed look at us and said, "Is this the medical fantasy room?" And in unison we shouted: "No, no. This is reality."

Finally we got to the muscle man approach. One of the guys on the volunteer committee created a beautiful pamphlet of two muscle men joining the vaccine study and we handed this right out in the street. We just grabbed the people, opened up a clinic wherever we were and hoped that they would go from us on the street into the clinic. The main thing was to get that blood test. Meantime, of course, we were still going to all the clubs and all the usual organizations, and people from these groups were joining in as volunteers. So there was this kind of reaching out everywhere and it was really quite wonderful and extraordinary.

But the biggest job I had to do was to convince the gay community leaders that participation in this trial would enhance their self-image. Once that was picked up people were very responsive and helping in the hepatitis B vaccine program became their personal gesture toward their gay identity and that of the movement. It was most moving for me to get that kind of commitment.

But still Szmuness was not satisfied. The day he told John Morrison that they simply had to work harder and sign up fifteen hundred men, is a day Morrison prefers to forget. He couldn't argue the point, but he thought of his twenty volunteers who showed up week in week out, recruiting at all hours, in the cold and the rain, working harder than at any other time in their lives, ten to fourteen hours a day, six days a week, enrolling in the Bloodmobile or on the streets or in the clinics, until all hours – talking, persuading, informing, beguiling. Everyone who dropped by was given the spiel, and if in a week's time, the test showed a man he was free of infection the persuasion would begin. Were they interested in the trial? Would they join in? If so could they promise, *please*, to follow through to the end? Exhausting it certainly was, but in one way it was also fun, John Morrison says, because most of the people in the study had a good education, many were professionals, and their questions were challenging. They took great interest not only in such small points as to whether the injection would hurt, but in larger ones such as how the vaccine was made. Since John Morrison's primary job was to gain total commitment, and he knew that only if the men really understood what was going on would he get it, he tried to show the volunteers how the study was as much theirs as the Blood Center's, that they had an important role not only for Greenwich Village, New York, but for the rest of the world. He forced them to make the leap from themselves to their community, and then to the wider family of humanity. Mostly this worked and they signed up. When it didn't, he tried badgering.

By the end of the drive 1,083 men had agreed to take part and signed the consent form, but to find them, the staff had screened more than 10,000 people.

Having signed up this small army, the recruiters now had to keep their recruits in line using any means from persuasion to nagging. Each participant would have three injections of vaccine or placebo – the first shot, then the second one a month later, and a booster injection six months after the first. But this was not all. Blood specimens would be taken regularly, at three-monthly intervals, during the first year and then at eighteen months, and finally at twenty-four months. Even this might not be all. If there were any abnormalities in a man's blood, then further samples would be required, and it was the recruiter's responsibility, and especially that of the Project's manager, to see that the protocols were rigidly adhered to by every single person.

The full force of Wolf Szmuness's character now surfaced: his steely persistence; his impatience with irritating persons or frustrating circumstances; his roar of anger; his authoritarian tactics; his total unwavering commitment; his unrelenting hard work; his satisfied silence, which at first they could not read; his short snappy "Nao"; his slow smile of pleasure. All these revealed someone concentrating every ounce of scientific experience, every fiber of personal being on the most important task he would ever undertake. There was no place for waverers or doubters, no room for anyone who was not prepared to throw himself unstintingly into months of exhausting activity. People who complained that they were having a hard time, putting in long hours in tough circumstances, were firmly blown away by Szmuness's "Pff! I've been in Siberia" and there was no convincing comeback to that.

Cladd Stevens played a pivotal role between the man from Siberia and the men in Greenwich Village. She rapidly adapted to Szmuness's demanding ways, to his autocratic style of running the program; she had to. In spite of the ideal image of science, there is rarely anything very democratic about the leadership of a major scientific operation, especially when its leader, whether American or Central European, has a clear vision and an obsessive determination to carry out a preconceived plan. But Stevens learned greatly from Szmuness and now says he taught her so well that in future her standards will always have his as a measure. As her confidence and understanding of epidemiology and Wolf increased more and more, she would stand up, argue back, wait, and then maneuver to calm things down. At times this was very necessary. Compassionate and imaginative though Szmuness was, his understanding of people was often faulty, perhaps because he had no time. A warm, gentle, and caring woman, Stevens endeared herself to the gay community by stepping into every breach, seeing that no one was ever exploited, and smoothing ruffled feathers. Stevens was not free of worry, however.

We were really going into unknown territory. First of all, we were asking a lot of the participants and we didn't know what their response would be. Then, the vaccine was experimental, and though it had already been given to several hundred people in the trials for safety and immune response, this was the first time it had been used on thousands. I was very tense about this. I worried we might even have a major reaction – an anaphylactic shock – when a person experiences an instantaneous, and often fatal, immunological response. So as a kind of insurance policy I insisted that everyone involved in actually administering the vaccine take a course in cardiopulmonary resuscitation. So we all trooped down to the Red Cross and practiced on *Resuscie Annie*, their plastic model. Wolf told me I was overreacting, but still I was really nervous as I watched the first volunteer receive his injection.

The volunteer was Rick Sardovsky, a gay physician and an active worker at the Gay Men's Health Project, who had his own reasons for volunteering to be first:

Sure, I was a little bit nervous, but knowing that at least two hundred physicians at the University Hospital in New York Medical Center had taken the injection before helped a great deal. It was important to me because I am a physician who works at a major medical center here in New York City, and research is the major way physicians can get ahead in the academic situation here. This was an opportunity to participate in a spectacularly well designed trial, which had on its advisory board several of the most renowned hepatologists, like Bob McCollum and Saul Krugman, and hematologists, like Scott Swisher, and epidemiologists from the whole country. So it was a chance to meet them, learn how they work, and participate in a project in which we were all deeply involved.

Stevens watched Rick Sardovsky tensely. The needle slid in and then out and with a cheery comment the first volunteer to be "stuck" went merrily on his way.

Soon they were mired in the daily sequences of the trial. As the weeks turned into months and the seasons of the next year and a half marched across the city, the exacting routine went on and on. Now Szmuness drove himself and his staff even harder, and the effects rippled home where Maya Szmuness strove to provide a calm, unruffled, still center of support. "He was incredibly tense throughout the whole eighteen months – very excited," she remembers. "Walking on the beach, talking, watching

TV news, eating his supper, he would interrupt everything – his mind always busy with hepatitis. I think for the whole eighteen months every half hour he would stand up, walk around, then write something down before he forgot."

He never relaxed an inch. Periodically John Morrison would meet with Szmuness, sometimes alone, sometimes with the advisory board, and Szmuness's reaction was always the same: "This trial is a disaster!" Morrison was to hear that sentence so often that now, when he visits the Blood Center, the secretaries take one look at him and chant "This is a disaster." He heard the phrase every day and the entire staff heard it every month. They would sit around a table, during their regular meetings, with sandwich lunches and wait for Szmuness to start, always in the same way. At first some people would be on the verge of baffled anger, and others would ask "Why?" and "How?" and Szmuness would counter: "Why has this person not come in for a while? Why has this person dropped out completely? Why is this person late on his test?"

Whenever volunteers disappeared, a "Lost to Follow-Up Form" had to be submitted on which all attempts to contact them, whether by telephone, mail, telegram, or visit, had to be recorded with the dates. Over and over the telephone call would be placed, "Look, John (or Pete, or Ed, or Stan), the records show you didn't show up for your third injection (or follow-up blood test). It's really important that you stick to the schedule. Please come in tomorrow." Monitoring the spectrum of activities from recruitment to follow-up, Szmuness constantly nagged, but eventually the staff began to see what he wanted and why – total adherence to the time-table because the trial was strictly a one-time event.

As time passed, Morrison began to guess where gaps might appear, would move to fill them, and have the information ready before Szmuness asked questions. No one blew up under the pressure and nobody threw in the towel. For as they came to understand just what a clinical trial involved, the fact that haunted Szmuness became apparent: *there would be no second chance*. If the trial were done improperly, if the vaccine seemed to be only marginally effective even though in reality it was highly effective, if because people were lost to follow-up, the extent of protection seemed low, then that was that. The trial could never be repeated. Not only would such repetition be unethical, it would be impractical too. The result would stick and the ambiguous reputation of the first hepatitis B vaccine would hover forever as an unwelcome miasma. Szmuness's life work, together with the efforts of all these people, would melt away as the whispered rumor spread through the scientific community: "It was a sloppy piece of work."

So they kept going. Then Szmuness increased the number of follow-up blood tests and sent a letter to the volunteers to tell them. Now they had to persuade over a thousand people to accept yet another schedule and adhere to it. Morrison was appalled, but since he couldn't really say, "I don't want to do this," he wrote a memorandum in which he carefully emphasized the cost and the extra workload for the laboratory and recruiting personnel. Apprehensively he took this into Szmuness, who read it slowly and carefully. Then he looked up and with an enormous smile he said: "You think you're going to get around me. But no, John, I want these blood tests." They both laughed but Szmuness got his way.

The extra tests were necessary because Szmuness needed to extract every ounce of information from this trial, and once again he had only one chance. Certainly the trial would reveal whether or not the vaccine afforded protection against hepatitis B. But if it did, he also wanted to know how quickly the antibodies formed; whether these increased with each successive injection, and how long their effects lasted. He needed, that is, to know whether the vaccine could be given in one shot that gives lifetime protection, or whether regular booster injections would be needed. So after the three vaccinating jabs into the 1,083 volunteers, a further 6,332 follow-up visits and blood samples were also scheduled. The demands on the gay population were not confined to the demanding protocols of the trial. Someone had to supply vaccine, so quantities of blood serum were needed for present and future supplies. Three hundred carrier donors, paid fifty dollars a time, gave serum and some did so as many as one hundred and fifty times during the eighteen-month period – a figure that was only possible because their red blood cells were returned to them.

One day, about a year into the trial, John Morrison walked into Szmuness's office and, on hearing the familiar words, calmly looked him straight in the eye and simply smiled. For a long, silent moment, Szmuness returned the look and then he, too, began to laugh: things *were* going very well. Yet still he kept up the pressure. His staff may have worked harder for him than any of them ever had for anyone else, but they would do so again any time, they say. His insistence on everyone matching his own impeccable standards could have provoked a disaster, but it did not, for his staff loved him even though they were totally exasperated at times, when he seemed quite intolerable, unappreciative, unreasonably demanding, and impossibly exacting. Like a bull about to charge, down would go his head, and they would brace themselves for criticism.

It was his credibility that saved him. Szmuness may have been meticulous in setting out rules and insisting that they be followed to the letter, but he followed those rules himself. He may have been an impossibly strict disciplinarian, but he brought the same discipline to his own time and work, wedding his formidable critical skills to those statistical techniques that gave weight to his scientific understanding and intuition. He never tried to dispose either of facts that didn't fit or situations that were difficult. Although he was often emotional, he never gave an emotional response to a scientific observation, and when emotional responses came, they derived, the staff quickly sensed, more from deep-seated anxieties than anything else. Tough he most certainly was, but as they look back at what was required, they see that toughness of all kinds was a factor in the trial's ultimate success or failure.

He was an alchemist. A formidable scientific personality and visionary imagination created a magical atmosphere where everyone felt an integral part of a unique venture. "I think the scientific aspects of the trial," says Morrison, "the goals and the realities, and how it was pursued, were extraordinary. Obviously very stringent, very careful, very precise. The compliance, too, of the gay community was extraordinary. Those are the two magic things that brought it right across." And it was Szmuness who molded the amalgam.

But inexorably, pressures began to build on him, stemming from the imperatives built into clinical trials. He knew the rules and was not unprepared for the problems. He could have chanted the commandments carved onto the tablets of all clinical trials: "Thou shalt not depart from the protocols until the trial has run its full course." "Thou shalt not treat a person who becomes ill with your trial remedy even if you think it might help." "Thou shalt not reveal what a patient has received." If these commandments are broken, data are obscured and years of work wasted. So fervently are these imperatives upheld that Sinclair Lewis, in his famous novel, *Arrowsmith*, was able to make their violation the climax of his story, without stretching credulity or realism one iota. (Martin Arrowsmith, sent to study a plague on a Caribbean island, tortured by his wife's death from the plague, treats a patient in his control group and, wracked with remorse, wonders how he can ever face his scientific mentor, Max Gottlieb, again.)

In anticipation of the problems such imperatives engender, Szmuness had appointed two external assessors to perform a vital dual function: his new friend, Saul Krugman, and his old correspondent, Dr. Robert McCollum, would guarantee the integrity of the trial and monitor its safety. If scientists have ways of finding out who has received what in a trial, then they can manipulate the results. The only total assurance of honesty is that the investigators *cannot* know who has received vaccine or placebo. The assessors alone held the code. They would be given the ID numbers of anyone who developed hepatitis B during the trial and would check the person's vaccine status. As safety officers they were in a position to protect all participants: they had the authority to stop the trial if they suspected that the vaccine was provoking the disease.

Everyone expected that, in the early stages, some cases of hepatitis B would occur among both placebo and vaccinated groups, for some people would already be incubating the virus when they signed up. Even if the vaccine protected, it would be some four months and two injections later before the immune response became total, so again, the disease might show up in some vaccine recipients. No one was seriously perturbed when reports of hepatitis came in early, not even Szmuness, who worried easily. One volunteer became sick, was hospitalized, and the Blood Center paid the bills even though his illness had nothing to do with the trial. But news of the free medical care spread quickly, and this was good public relations. The Blood Center was seen to be sticking by its promises, which was important because volunteers were still being recruited.

Then one Sunday in September 1979, a serious crisis erupted. Jimmy, a waiter, was found unconscious and on the floor was his ID card. Soon the screaming sirens and screeching brakes reverberated round the unconscious man as he was rushed to Bellevue Hospital. Quickly doctors diagnosed his condition: he was suffering from fulminating hepatitis and in the early stages of its terminal phase. They felt that they really must know just what kind of case they had under their hands. Bellevue was Krugman's hospital, but he was out of town; so too was Szmuness. Traced to Geneva, where they were both attending a conference, they said to call Bob McCollum. He, too, was not at home, but tracked to the tennis court at his country club.

He called Saul Krugman, and they decided he should break the code. So McCollum unlocked the drawer on the right-hand side of his office desk, retrieved the written key, and broke the code. It was not until the trial was over, however, that Szmuness and Stevens were to learn that Jimmy was a placebo recipient and that the vaccine could in no way have been associated with his disease. He survived.

This was a rare case, but physicians regularly telephoned, insisting on being told the vaccine status of patients who had contracted hepatitis. The information was never given, but the staff had regularly to cope with angry comments: "I don't care about the results of your God-damn trial: what about my patient?"

This was mild compared with what was to come. Once the trial was under way Wolf Szmuness and Cladd Stevens sought approval to do something else. Was it possible that repeated injections of the vaccine could be useful as therapy as well as protection? Sixteen hepatitis B carriers volunteered to receive twice as many injections of the vaccine as anyone else. Each man would receive one injection of vaccine every month for six months and it would be a simple test with no placebos. The men felt they had nothing to lose: the vaccine was safe, their medical future bleak, and if this did work, it would be a bonus for the scientists and a miracle for carriers. Several months into this trial one man developed non-A non-B hepatitis. Four weeks later, when Wolf was out of town, another man in the group developed the same thing. Stevens, also on her way out of town for a few days, left a note on Szmuness's desk reporting yet another case. "When I returned a few days later," she recalls, "all kinds of uproar had broken loose."

Szmuness was anxious. Could the vaccine be provoking non-A non-B hepatitis, and worse, was there a similar pattern developing in the main trial that no one had yet noticed? He asked Saul Krugman, as a matter of urgency, to check out the occurrence of non-A non-B cases in the main trial, in all recipients. If he found that more people in the vaccinated group were succumbing, would he call immediately but tell Szmuness *only* that. Krugman was soon back with the figures: three hundred people had, by then, received injections, there were fourteen possible cases of non-A non-B hepatitis and of these eleven had occurred among vaccinated people, two among the placebos, and one diagnosis was dubious.

Szmuness considered this information carefully. Since half the main trial group was receiving the vaccine and half the placebo, on the surface the flare-up of non-A non-B hepatitis appeared to be a vaccine-associated event. At this moment, he thought he faced disaster.

Was something wrong with the vaccine, possibly contamination? This was no theoretical fear, contamination having been suspected in one vaccine batch made by the National Institutes of Health, though never in Merck's. His instinct was to stop the trial. Stevens returned in the middle of the consequent uproar. Szmuness placed a conference call to all parties, the government in the form of the National Institutes of Health authorities, the producers of the vaccine, Merck, and the safety officers, Saul Krugman and Bob McCollum. He outlined the facts and everyone began talking, but eventually it came down to, "You're the principal investigator. Whatever you decide to do, we'll agree."

In an interview some years later Szmuness explained his reasoning:

I wanted to stop the trial at once because the basic principle of any clinical experiment is not to do harm to the participants. Their interests are always of the first importance. You should not – you don't have the right to – harm them. So my first inclination was to see what happened with the vaccine and through that find the cause of this non-A, non-B hepatitis outbreak. We weren't the only people to notice it. Government scientists who worked independently with another vaccine were seeing several cases; some were occurring among monks in Texas. So I felt only if we found a reasonable explanation could we then continue.

Of course I sought advice, but as frequently happens in a situation like this, everybody gave advice but no one wanted to take the responsibility of stopping the trial. Only Saul Krugman, with his special type of wisdom, that of an excellent scientist with a long experience not only in science, but in the suffering of being a scientist,* stepped in. "You know Wolf," he said, "Let us take the responsibility together. I am close to seventy-five; you also are not a young man and we are both doing the right thing – an important thing – and I think we will survive this."

Another person who was very helpful was Aaron Kellner. I told him first that everything I was about to discuss was in total confidence. Nothing must be said until a decision had been made, in case the matter got to the newspapers.

His fears were totally understandable. It would have been calamitous had the trial stopped: the particular vaccine could never be used again, for it would have the reputation of causing disease. Worse, its reputation would cloak all future hepatitis B vaccines and progress might be set back by a decade. Yet, if Szmuness allowed the trial to proceed, people might die, he would be branded a murderer, and there was, he feared, a real possibility that he would be jailed.

Recounting this conversation, Szmuness emphasizes how wise, gentle, and full of common sense Kellner had been. His advice was to wait a few weeks and see how things worked out; he, Kellner, had worked for thirty years in this area and in the initial stages there always were apparent problems. But Szmuness was not easily reassured.

Szmuness's anxiety was not irrational overdramatization. "On the one hand," Aaron Kellner comments, "he was remembering his experiences in Russia. But on the other hand, the sudden termination of the swine flu vaccination program a few years back was very much on people's minds. The effect on one's personal life and career can be devastating, for the public is unforgiving about things like that, even if people are innocent of any wrongdoing."

* Krugman had been bitterly attacked, not for his early experiments on a hepatitis B vaccine, but for the fact that mentally retarded children were involved.

Wolf was concerned for everyone's reputation, actually: if something disastrous happened it would also reflect back on Merck, and the gay community, too. Yet his choices seemed stark: he was in a no-win situation. He could kill the trial or take a dreadful risk. "If I am wrong," he repeated to Kellner, "I'll go to jail. My scientific career will be in shreds and I will be faced with an enormous amount of litigation as well." For even though a consent form is a *consent* form it actually does not eliminate risks of legal suits should anyone become seriously ill.

Kellner, Cladd Stevens, and Saul Krugman together, all reassured and teased him: he must wait and see how the situation developed; if the problems were real they'd pay the lawyers, take care of Maya, bring him food and flowers in jail; Stevens said she'd go in too and would plan in advance what work they would do there together. They would, Kellner assured him, tap the best lawyers in the United States, and finally Saul Krugman volunteered to come to jail too. Szmuness eventually joined in the joshing even though it was all too near the bone. Finally, with great trepidation, he decided that the trial should go on; yet, as with the visit to Russia, he rested his confidence ultimately on the same two people "in whom," he said, "I have one hundred percent trust."

But there's a fine line between risk and judgment, as Bob McCollum admitted when asked if he would have stopped the trial then or if Jimmy the waiter had been a vaccine recipient.

In theory, you make your decisions on a logical, cold, and quite legitimate basis. So, one would say, go on. On the other hand, both conscience and emotion *do* play a part and inevitably *have* to play a part. It's a very, very fine line indeed, between saying "I have the authority so I'll make the decision and live by the consequences," and allowing your personal feelings – which include the fine weight of your judgment and experience – to call a halt. You would be making a decision that some would consider outrageously arbitrary but others would consider the only possible decision. In the end, of course, we would take such a decision only on the basis of a pattern and we had to wait for that to emerge. However, while waiting, we'd know full well that if things were going wrong, others would be receiving perhaps their third injections of a material that was causing trouble.

Afterward Dr. Bob Purcell, of the National Institutes of Health, came up with an explanation for the scare. Clearly all the volunteers were being exposed to, and some were catching, both hepatitis B and the non-A non-B form. Since at the time there was no blood test for non-A non-B hepatitis, any blood sample from someone with both infections showed only B. Unprotected patients receiving the placebo were catching dual infections but showing only B in their blood tests. Because patients receiving vaccine were protected against B and so would only contract and show non-A non-B hepatitis, this form was bound to appear in higher numbers in the vaccine group.

Everything calmed down again. The weeks slid by and the seasons swung again. By Easter 1980 the end was in sight. The project staff at the Blood Center was checking the records and making lists of those in the clinical trial who had developed hepatitis B. There were one hundred and sixty cases.

One month later, in June 1980, Cladd Stevens left for work early. It was no ordinary day. Once at the Blood Center she and her three colleagues crammed into Wolf Szmuness's tiny office. Two were tense, but two were trying to maintain the poker faces that they had been wearing now for six months. Saul Krugman and Bob McCollum had met regularly to look at the figures and three months before the code was officially broken the patterns were telling them the answer, even six months before that they would have bet money on the result. But as they had gone about their business they had given no clue as to what they knew.

Stevens sat down opposite Krugman, Szmuness opposite McCollum. Stevens had the assembled sheets of paper listing the code numbers of the people in the trial who had contracted hepatitis during its course. Krugman and McCollum had the same list too, but alongside their numbers was the word "vaccine" or the word "placebo." Stevens called off a number and the two men said "placebo." Then she called off another and again the chorus said "placebo"; yet another and once more "placebo."

"It got to be very, very monotonous," she recalls, "and then the more monotonous it got, the more exciting it got. Finally, we looked at each other and said, 'do you think we need bother with a statistical analysis?', it was so obvious what was going on."

They sensed that they were home and dry within five minutes. They felt that the litany "placebo, placebo, placebo" would never end, nor did it. As the excitement of Stevens and Szmuness mounted, the smiles of Krugman and McCollum broadened. In perhaps the most daring gesture of his scientific life, Wolf Szmuness had already bought the champagne, and Aaron Kellner was called in to help finish off the bottle.

The cork popped, the bubbles fizzed, the glasses clinked. From high excitement they descended into abysmal chaos. Of course they had to get a whole series of more sophisticated analyses. They had to call up the results from the computer and look at the statistical patterns, for from the graphs they had to *see* that the protection the figures revealed could be legitimately interpreted to one cause and that one *only* – the vaccine. They wanted this knowledge right there and then. But computers have no sense of occasion and this one went "down." Wolf Szmuness seethed with frustration but couldn't order the machine to perform.

A few days later, they broke the code again to the Advisory Board. By then rumors of a major success were buzzing around the Blood Center. It was supposed to have been top secret but, like all such secrets, it leaked. Saul Krugman had asked three outside doctors, all with distinguished experience in hepatitis, to examine the clinical records of every case of hepatitis B and say whether the diagnosis had been correct, for once again any ambiguity here would be a point of attack by critics. Thus all cases were eventually diagnosed three times: by Cladd Stevens and Dan William, by Bob McCollum and Saul Krugman, and finally by the outside doctors. They completely agreed with all the previous diagnoses and so the code was formally broken again. Once more the litany was chanted: "Placebo, placebo, placebo."

One member of the advisory board, Dr. Scott Swisher, a distinguished hematologist, excitedly recalls their triumph in a wonderful mixture of metaphors:

Everyone had a look on their faces of the fox eating the grapes. It was like the race track when you can't lose because you're betting on the best horse. The expectation was that the result would be a real plum and it was. There was a level of quiet exaltation that was a joy to see and be part of. Wolf was making a valiant effort – and succeeding pretty well – in playing the role of a cool, objective scientist, reporting his results. But those who knew him, sensed his excitement and his personal satisfaction, but not in terms of *his* accomplishment alone. There was a feeling of great pride and humility.

Szmuness knew that Merck had a major immunoprotective agent of enormous value for the whole world. Constantly he spoke of the teamwork, of the mutual feelings of respect and consideration that had been built up between himself and the gay community, and how these had important values in themselves, over and above the success of the vaccine. He talked about his own personal transformation. He, too, was feeling better about these people in a human and a social sense.

John Morrison recalls the crazy wildness of that day, though his memories are thoroughly intoxicated, for he had come down with scarlet fever but had no idea what was wrong. He was swollen, uncomfortable, and covered with a rash, his hands in such bad shape that he couldn't hold anything. Since it was such an important occasion he felt obliged to dress in a decent all-weather suit, a torture device, he says, "that doesn't keep you warm in winter and is impossibly hot in summer." His temperature was way up and the results sent it higher.

The staff remembers the elated satisfaction of that day. Szmuness, restless with excitement, kept popping in and out of the committee room. Sometimes he would come to where they waited, just look at them, not say a word, put his head down in that characteristic fashion, and disappear, but sometimes he spoke: "It's going good. It's going good." They had suspected that things *were* good at their last meeting, when Szmuness had opened the proceedings and with resignation they had waited for the familiar complaint, but, instead, he said, "This is a beautiful trial!" Some had wanted to cry, some to laugh, but all recollect a rising tide of warmth and love for this man who had carried, badgered, bullied, sustained, and led them to a triumphant climax, a result of which they are all so proud that each has said: "In the future, I shall boast: 'I took part in the hepatitis B vaccine trial'."

They had every reason to boast. Of the 1,083 people who received the first injection, 1,040 (96.5 percent) showed up for the second. By the end of the trial, 40 percent of the volunteers had been expected to drop out; only 15.4 percent did. After the three injections 6,332 follow-up visits were scheduled and a staggering 5,774 – that is, 91.2 percent – took place. The performance of the vaccine was equally dramatic: it was shown to be 81 percent effective in provoking antibodies in those who received at least one injection. In those who received all three injections, 96 percent developed antibodies against the virus. Only 3.4 percent in this group developed hepatitis B, in contrast to 27 percent of the placebo group, and this mostly occurred within five months of the trial's start, so these people were harboring the infection before the trial ever began. A significant reduction in the incidence of the disease was observed in the group only seventy-five days into the trial, which suggests that, as with rabies vaccine, protection is effective *even* if the person has already been exposed. Such an effect was a magnificent – and unsuspected – bonus. Overall, the vaccine was shown to be 92.3 percent effective in protecting high-risk individuals against hepatitis B: these findings are of an order of magnitude that has never been equaled in any other vaccine trial, either before or since.

As the data and clinical histories were analyzed, other results began to spin off. It became clear that hepatitis A, too, has a much higher attack rate in gay men than in others, but no one knows why. Unpleasant though hepatitis B may be, it appears to be a self-limiting disease in most Western societies, but, again, no one knows why. Because it is self-limiting, though 160 out of the 1,083 trial volunteers did become ill with hepatitis B, only three needed to be hospitalized. Finally, the Blood Center has a unique blood bank. It comprises first, the sera of those men in the study who became ill, with their blood samples stored sequentially, beginning when they were noninfectious, right through to illness and cure. But it also has the blood sera of over thirteen thousand gay men, three thousand who took part in the baseline studies and the ten thousand who were screened for the trial, and this blood was banked at Szmuness's insistence. One day, worrying that he was pushing himself too hard, his wife anxiously asked him, "Why are you bothering with all this?" With imaginative foresight Szmuness replied, "Because one day another disease may erupt and we'll need this material." When AIDS did indeed erupt a few years later Cladd Stevens and the scientists turned with gratitude and relief to this bank of blood for the unique clues it provides.

The gay community were as elated as the scientists. Their co-operation had been unstinting, and they took the keenest interest, and still do, in the progress of our battle against hepatitis. John Morrison says with pride: "I know over a thousand people now. They stop me all over the city and say, 'Hi, John. I was in the trial. We did a good job there. What's happening now? How's Cladd? What's Dr. Szmuness up to these days?'"

Two weeks after the code was broken, Szmuness threw a big party for everyone who had been involved, with more champagne and many toasts. They loved Szmuness again that day. He was very modest but it was no false modesty, for he knew precisely the importance of their success. Yet he shuffled around, elated at their joint success, yet embarrassed at the same time.

Success was due both to the existence of a superb vaccine and to the design and execution of the trial. This was not only the most complex ever in the history of medicine, but was also the most impeccable. Earlier trials – such as those held in the 1950s for the polio vaccine, which were some of the first controlled, double-blind field trials – had never given similarly clear-cut results. This was because the incidence of paralytic polio was far lower than the incidence of hepatitis B. It was also because polio trials had been done in several populations, in several parts of the country, at different times, in different settings, so that many ambiguities inevitably slid into the final results.

With his trial, however, Wolf Szmuness had total control, one willingly granted, of a compact, high-risk population, in one geographic spot, for eighteen months. His genius had been in recognizing that the gay community held all the necessary elements for success. In one imaginative leap, he had perceived both the extent of the problem and its solution. He had worked out in advance what data could be derived from the trial in the time available, had listed the myriad pieces of additional information that it could be made to yield, and designed it in such a way that these *were* yielded. Certainly other people had considered using the gay population in a clinical trial, but none had ever done so. Only Szmuness, in a series of logical, beautifully designed steps, began at the beginning and marched through to the triumphant end.

The scientific paper that communicated the results to the wider scientific community created a sensation. It first appeared on October 9, 1980, in the prestigious *New England Journal of Medicine,* where every scientist-clinician yearns to be published. Nine authors were listed, beginning with Szmuness and ending with Aaron Kellner, and included not only the two gay physicians, Dan William and Richard Sardovsky, but John Morrison, Cladd Stevens, Ed Harley, and two other members of the New York Blood Center, Edith Zang and William Oleszko. The lead editorial in the issue described the trial as "immaculate in design and execution." The equally prestigious scientific journal, *Nature,* published from London, also covered the story on the same day. Emphasizing both the unusual source of the vaccine and Szmuness's meticulous organization, the editor described the trial as "a milestone in the annals of preventive medicine." The Blood Center held a press conference and shortly after, Szmuness presented the results to his scientific peers and, for the second time in his life, received a standing ovation. The seal of approval on the vaccine's success came a year later, on November 17, 1981, when the U.S. Food and Drug Administration announced it had approved the licensing of the first vaccine against hepatitis B. The fifteen-year time span between the discovery of the virus and final governmental approval for a protective vaccine is the shortest ever recorded in the history of any infectious disease whatever.

Asked in 1981, "How was this short time lag possible?", Wolf Szmuness replied:

There were four elements and if any one had been missing, success would have been impossible. First, the tools, both intellectual and technological, suddenly became very sophisticated; second, a large group of dedicated people – some who'd spent years working on hepatitis, some sufferers from hepatitis – cooperated on the problem; third, support came from the government through the backing of the National Institutes of Health (NIH), and finally there were regular injections of both private and public money. The regularity was far more important than the actual amounts.

"So what are you going to do next," I asked. There were several things. For a start, the people who took part in the original trial had to be closely monitored to determine how long the protection lasts. Other trials were also set up. Similar trials with male homosexuals but now using only half the dose of vaccine, were repeated in Atlanta and in five other cities around the United States. Trials were also conducted within two other groups: hospital medical staffs, known to be at high risk from hepatitis B, and 1,270 patients and other key medical staff within selected renal dialysis units. The kidney patients were under great stress, for twice a week they had to be dialyzed for six hours, and a very high mortality rate existed in the group. Ten percent of such people die every year; the death of any participant in the trial, for whatever reason, had to be checked and analyzed. Since deaths were occurring among the dialysis patients all the time, this was a very distressing period for Szmuness and his colleagues.

But most important of all were the global aspects of the disease – the area closest to Szmuness's heart. Trials were started in the Kangwane region of the Eastern Transvaal in South Africa with Swazi mothers and babies, a population that has large recurring pools of infection. Set up with the same meticulous planning as the original ones, these trials tackled the truly severe problems including, ultimately, that of liver cancer. These trials were watched with care, for the mothers acquire hepatitis, not by sexual activity or accidental needle pricks, but from general infection. The children catch it directly from their parents, sometimes immediately at birth, or possibly even in utero. So the scientists needed to answer such questions as, "Can babies be protected by the vaccine and if so, how long does the effect last and is the vaccine effective if given soon after birth?" Giving the vaccine to newborns is a race against time. Their immune system takes three months to become effective, but the hepatitis B virus takes the same time to incubate and become infective.

By 1984 the results were in; they look impressive. The vaccine seems to be winning the race against the virus, and even newborn babies start to make antibodies. Though it is not yet known how long protection lasts, it is already apparent that hepatitis B vaccine will one day be included in those routine shots that already protect babies from diseases like polio or measles. Thus we can reasonably expect that the large pool of infection will be reduced; so, in the long term, we can anticipate a worldwide reduction in liver cancer. The hepatitis B vaccine truly is our first anticancer vaccine.

Eradicating hepatitis B from the face of the earth was Szmuness's ultimate dream, and he fervently believed this was possible. When he said in 1981, "For the first time in my life I am truly happy," he meant two things. At one level this was a simple statement of fact. At another it stemmed from the possibility of an achievable vision. Szmuness was a man possessed by a burning desire to eliminate suffering and sickness, a desire that possibly stemmed from the unhappiness of his early life. But he was not a simple do-gooder whose vision was determined by wishful thinking. He knew that if you are to eliminate sickness, reduce suffering, conquer disease, it has to be done with one solid fact laid upon another and another and eventually success will come. It was, both Saul Krugman and Aaron Kellner constantly emphasized, in that method that lay the keys to his triumph.

Aaron Kellner believes this experiment has influenced medicine permanently: "This trial was both a milestone and a classic. It was a milestone since this was the first time that we had tools to prevent and conquer a major disease. It was a classic in the way Wolf did it, the sensitive and meticulous planning, the solid way in which the data were gathered, the unimpeachable findings. It is now *such* a classic that it may be unethical to do any other trial differently."

So often is this meticulousness mentioned when researchers and clinicians speak of the study, that when I asked Wolf Szmuness "What is the most important quality in a scientist?" his reply took me by surprise. "Imagination. Not so much hard work, but imagination. Without it you will never be a good scientist." Commented Kellner,

Well, Wolf could discern differences that eluded others. It was the mixture – the use of his imagination and the quantitative analysis of the differences he saw – that made him the genius he was. And look at the consequences. Most physicians influence the lives of a few hundred – at the most a few thousand – people. Some fortunate ones can influence the lives of a few million. It is the rare physician, who, like Wolf Szmuness, is given the grace to touch the lives of billions of people, those living on this planet and generations yet unborn.

He will receive this grace, for already major vaccination programs are underway in countries like Hong Kong, Japan, Singapore, Korea. In Taiwan a national campaign against hepatitis B has been mounted and, starting with babies at risk, the government expects to have universal vaccination in the whole population in ten years. The protection of the vaccine is underpinned with the use of disposable syringes and a campaign to persuade people to use disposable chopsticks.

There is still a long way to go before Szmuness's dream is realized. A massive worldwide campaign to eradicate hepatitis B is still some way off. The question "Can it be done?" is becoming "Who will pay?" Protection presently costs between $75 and $100 and by anyone's standards this is far too high. Another difficulty is that the demands of the homosexual population are very great. Carrier volunteers from the study have been recruited as the source and are more than happy to help, but it would be much better if the vaccine were not so absolutely dependent on human beings. Sustained efforts will always be necessary both to keep the volunteers motivated and to ensure that no infectious contaminants slip in.

Though these problems are not insuperable, other, cheaper, sources of vaccine are far more than just a gleam in the eye. The newest techniques of recombinant DNA biology are providing one alternative. One genetically engineered vaccine has already been tested in chimpanzees and its certification is expected. It will cost a mere ten dollars a shot. Merck, too, has developed a genetically engineered vaccine that has gone through successful trials in laboratory animals and preliminary ones in human volunteers. In both cases the vaccine confers strong protection. Synthetic vaccines are also undergoing tests, and these vaccines are prototypes for future ones. No live viruses, or even bits of them, are used; instead, the necessary molecules are artificially assembled. Not only are they safer, but in the end will be considerably cheaper.

Doctors Geoffrey Smith, Michael Mackett, and Bernard Moss of the National Institute of Allergy and Infectious Diseases in Bethesda, Maryland, have done something stunningly clever. Starting with *Vaccinia* virus, the form of cowpox that protected against smallpox, they have spliced into it the very gene that makes the surface protein of the hepatitis B virus – the molecule to which the immune system responds. This "hybrid virus" grows phenomenally well in cell culture and vast quantities can be made. When injected, rabbits respond by producing quantities of protective antibodies. So, the scientists conclude, such hybrid viruses have a great future and could bring down the costs of protection dramatically. The process not only is far cheaper than preparing serum from human carriers, but administering the vaccine would be as simple as smallpox was: no injections, merely a scratching of the skin.

Szmuness certainly anticipated all these developments. One cold December day in 1981 he asked to see me, and during the hour we spent together he spoke of how he wished to spend the next four years, of the work still to finish and of the time measured against the running out of the sands. His strength, determination, and visionary character were manifestly there, gentle and touching, tough and rueful, all at once. He told me that in the Soviet Union there exists a scientific index of forbidden work, just as in Rome there exists a Catholic index of forbidden books. To his amusement, he was still listed. His works had never been cited or quoted, either in the USSR or Poland, and it was not until the story of the hepatitis B vaccine was broadcast over the BBC World Service, as well as the Voice of America, that his compatriots in Poland and colleagues in the Soviet Union became aware of its existence. Then the requests for reprints flooded in and he received an invitation to visit Warsaw in the summer of 1981. He applied for a visa and everything seemed to be proceeding smoothly. But at the last moment the visa was refused, so he never returned to his native land.

He told me again that there were two happiest moments in his life which he would never forget, both in 1980: the first when he heard the unending litany of "placebo, placebo, placebo"; the second when one hundred and fifty people from all over the world came to the scientific meeting at the Blood Center and rose to him in a standing ovation.

Then his mood changed. "Last year," he said yet again, "was the happiest year of my life. But June, time goes so quickly and the doors of happiness close so swiftly. Is it not a tragedy," he suddenly burst out in a mixture of despair and savage anger, "that I have lung cancer? I always knew it was too good to last. I knew from the very beginning when that man pointed 'the long finger' at me."

We were speaking in Memorial Hospital, New York, and he was seriously ill. A few days later 1981 yielded to 1982. The seasons turned and spring had erupted in all its glory all over town when, one day, Aaron Kellner visited him at home. During the few moments the two men were alone Szmuness reached out, took Kellner's hands and with tears in his eyes asked, "Aaron, who will be my Kaddish?" Kaddish is the ancient prayer for the dead that traditionally is recited by sons in memory of parents. Kellner replied that his friends and colleagues, all would be his Kaddish. A few weeks later, in June 1982, they fulfilled that promise to the man who had unexpectedly appeared in their lives, stayed for a brief moment of time, and then just as swiftly vanished into the darkness.

3
The Three Valleys
of St. Lucia

Science is the art of the soluble.

P. B. Medawar, *The Art of the Soluble*

Politics is the art of the possible.

Prince Bismarck, in conversation with Meyer von Waldeck,
August 11, 1867

The slaves who were forcibly transported to the New World, their culture and identity smashed, took few things with them. Their diseases were one and along with their muscle power, these were profoundly to affect the countries emerging on the far side of the Atlantic. Yet over two hundred years later some of their descendants would make a unique contribution to the control of one serious disease, schistosomiasis, which afflicts millions all over the world. Their island, St. Lucia in the Caribbean, was to become a natural laboratory for an unusual experiment in medicine, and its people the willing objects of study. The experiment is now considered a classic. Lasting for sixteen years, it was a meticulously conducted research project, remarkably controlled, given that the laboratory was not a room but a country and its inhabitants not mice but human beings.

Wherever scientists do experiments, they try to reduce everything – whether questions, methods, or analyses – to as few and as simple as possible. They endeavor to eliminate all variables, so that both the experiment and its results can be reproduced, many times over if need be, by different scientists in different laboratories in different countries. It is through this repetition of questions, methods, and answers that the collective voice of science finally speaks. The question that the scientists on St. Lucia wanted to answer was very simple. Given that three proven methods for schistosomiasis control already existed, which was the best, the most practical, the most cost-effective, or most beneficial? The question may sound simple, but answering it meant solving a problem of great complexity. The disease is caused by a sophisticated parasite with a life-cycle partly spent inside complex human beings, whose social patterns resulted in large numbers inevitably catching the disease. Thus, as one of them put it, the scientists on St. Lucia faced "one helluva job."

Parasitic diseases have always been the most difficult to tackle and one index is medicine's total failure to make vaccines against them. The challenge is intensified when the parasites live deep in human tissues, away from the circulating cells of the immune system. A purgative dose can eliminate a worm living in the alimentary canal. Subtler pharmaceutical measures are needed for a parasite that burrows deep into liver or blood cells. And if that parasite is one that has evolved with such exquisite adaptiveness that it needs two hosts to complete its life cycle, the challenge becomes even more formidable. For while one can eliminate parasites from an individual patient, or a population, the secondary host persists, as a permanent bastion to be attacked, and so long as secondary hosts exist, reservoirs of parasites will remain. Thus no matter how good the therapy, the disease can never be eradicated.

Parasites may not be very engaging creatures, but they do represent the epitome of evolutionary ingenuity. For the life-cycle of a parasite with two hosts includes two stages adapted to the different bodily fluids of two different organisms. Moreover, the parasite also will have learned to evade its host's defense mechanisms. Judged by these criteria, the parasite the scientists were trying to control on St. Lucia is a gem.

The disease the parasite provokes, schistosomiasis, is a major global health problem affecting more than two hundred million people worldwide, a number equaled only by malaria. Half of the entire population of Egypt have the infection; so did one-third of St. Lucia's population of 120,000 people; so do one in twenty of the world's population. In seventy-four developing countries, wherever there are poor living conditions, lack of sanitation, and general poverty, up to six hundred million other people are at risk. Such numbers place an enormous burden on the health resources of the endemic countries, which none of them can afford, and as population pressure intensifies the demand for water, the numbers are expected to grow still further.

This chronic infection was once called *bilharzia* after the German scientist who discovered it, but today "schistosomiasis" is preferred for it identifies the water-borne, schizont worms responsible. A worm can lay huge numbers of eggs in the human body at frequent intervals, three hundred to three thousand at a time, and can keep this up, some estimates say, for up to twenty years, though the average time is six to eight. In two species the worms live in the veins around the small intestine; in the third, in those of the bladder and urinary tract. The disease is quantitative: the body reacts by surrounding the eggs with scar tissue. The more eggs there are, the more extensive the scars, and the worse the patient's symptoms and greater the loss of function. In serious infections the liver, spleen, and the lymph nodes become enormously enlarged, and if the loss of liver or bladder function becomes severe the patient will die.

One half of the life-cycle is spent in a human being, the other in a freshwater snail. Both animals become sick. In the heat of the sun, one snail discharges into the water nearly one hundred thousand tiny, free-swimming larvae, *cercariae*. These must find a human host quickly and each has only a few hours to do so. Usually people contract schistosomiasis very early in life, for as soon as children can toddle into a stream they are exposed to the microscopic, fork-tailed larvae that take less than two minutes to penetrate unbroken human skin. Once inside, the tail drops off and the biochemistry of the organism immediately changes: from being adapted to life in fresh water it can now survive in the salty environment of the human body. Burrowing through the muscles, the parasite is carried in the bloodstream throughout the body. Passing through the heart, then the lungs, it eventually comes to rest in the liver, where it matures and waits for a mate. If one appears, the pair join quite literally, then they migrate to their final habitat for a life of permanent egg production.

In the parasite's average lifespan of six years, one pair will produce 6.5 million eggs which, discharged into water via human excreta, provide a massive reservoir for another cycle of infection. Not all the eggs pass out; some are swept into the small blood vessels, where an inflammatory reaction sets in. Scar tissue is produced in the liver which can become as scarred as the liver of an alcoholic with cirrhosis. The spleen then enlarges and the patient develops varicose veins on the lower legs. Sometimes the veins around the esophagus burst and the patient bleeds massively or even dies from vomiting blood. But this only occurs in the later and severe stage of infection and is rare. There is some immune reaction to the worm's presence but never enough to penetrate the parasite's defenses and we still don't know why. The clinical effect is very precisely related to the number of eggs a patient harbors. Most people are infected with only a few worms and never develop a fatal infection.

One human being cannot infect another directly: only by going through a water snail can the parasite pass to another person. The eggs pass out of the excreta into the water and hatch into free-swimming embryos, *miracidia*. Once again this marks an extremely vulnerable point in the parasite's life-cycle, for these embryos must find freshwater snails. Only 1 percent of the egg larvae ever manage to penetrate snails, but this number is quite sufficient to maintain the chain of infection. Once infected, the snail too shows the disease. Its fleshy foot, lungs, and liver become distended as bunches of fast-dividing miracidial daughter cells divide, developing into the fork-tailed cercariae. Under the stimulus of the sun's heat these are shed into the water where they seek a human being, and the cycle starts over again.

Schistosomiasis is thus a disease of two different animals. The most dangerous snail is not one so ill that it dies, but one just a little sick which can discharge larvae continuously for nearly six months. The most dangerous human being for a snail is one who is constantly excreting eggs into the water. If human beings wish to control this disease they need to eradicate snails; if snails conducted control programs on schistosomiasis they would have to eradicate us.

Water is the key element that links us both in the vicious cycle. From the beginning of time snails have inhabited, and human beings have maintained close contact with water. We use it for washing, cooking, for our animals, and for recreation. We have gone to the rivers by necessity and have gone in company. Given only a brief contact with infected water, the average person runs only a minute risk. In the Nile delta, for example, the average person acquires only 1.6 worms per year. But heavy infections come to people caught up in those regular, traditional activities that take place alongside the irrigation canals of the Nile, or by the lakes of Tanzania, Uganda, the Sudan, Brazil, and other lands – children playing, women washing, men working. As the birthrate of the Third World nations increases, so the demand for water intensifies, leading to new, vital, irrigation schemes that vastly multiply the stretches of water that snails inhabit. With the construction of the Aswan dam in Egypt, this point has been illustrated with deadly precision: the Nile is more than two thousand miles long, but the irrigation ditches that now utilize the constant flow of water are fifteen times that length and Egypt's entire population, forty-five million people, lives along the Nile. Half now have schistosomiasis.

This then was the problem whose challenges the unique experiment would try to resolve. But why was St. Lucia chosen? The island lies just 14° north of the Equator between Martinique to the north and St. Vincent to the south. Exquisitely beautiful, spectacularly lush, it is small, twenty-seven miles long and fourteen wide, part of an extended volcanic chain running north-south through the Caribbean. In living memory peaks on both Martinique and St. Vincent have blown their tops with devastating effects, but St. Lucia has its own safety valve; at the southern end of the island a blow-hole near the surface relieves the pressure and amid the gases that are gently vented through the hole, hot sulfurous springs provide therapeutic baths.

The volcanic origins gave birth to a rugged island whose topography proved crucial to the experiment. The spine of the land is a mountain ridge covered by dense rain forest, a green canopy of tall trees, decorative ferns, dripping leaves, and soft undergrowth, inhabited by dangerous snakes and gaudy birds. The forests cover many of the peaks, from whose heights steep valleys have been cut by the streams. But so steep are the valleys, so high the hills, so small the footpaths that, to all intents and purposes, the valleys are completely isolated from each other; ecologically and socially there has been very little contact between their human communities.

One main road connects the international airport at the south to the capital, Castries, some ninety minutes' drive away to the northwest. Off the main road and into the interior, small tracks form a patchwork of narrow paths winding up hills, around corners, and down valleys. In the high hills the jungle predominates, but on the lower levels plantations of bananas and coconuts have been developed. Cocoa is grown also, and mangoes, avocados, coffee, oranges, grapefruit, sour-sop, yams, dasheen, breadfruit, and a tree with berries of superb protein – pigeon peas. Even in the dry season, December to April, rain falls every day. The clouds suddenly disintegrate into sweeping sheets that can drench you to the skin in under two minutes. The very same rain that produces the lush vegetation and magnificent crops also causes soil erosion, so most people now terrace their plots. Slope above slope the tiny gardens are worked and the produce swept into the markets every Saturday, when the people pile onto rickety minibuses and converge on Castries or Soufrière.

It sounds romantic, but it isn't, for the picturesque beauty masks desperate poverty. In the hinterland the houses are simple wooden shacks, supported on stilts above the mud. For generations, sugar had been the main crop, but in the last century a switch was made to bananas. This change affected both human and natural ecology – and, the scientists were to discover, – schistosomiasis too. The people were forced higher up the hillsides and their "slash, burn, grow, move on" techniques destroyed patches of the rain forest and provoked soil loss. The change did have one advantage, though: sugar needed vast numbers of people to harvest the cane and these were usually slaves or, after slavery was abolished in 1893, indentured servants. But anyone can grow bananas and most St. Lucians

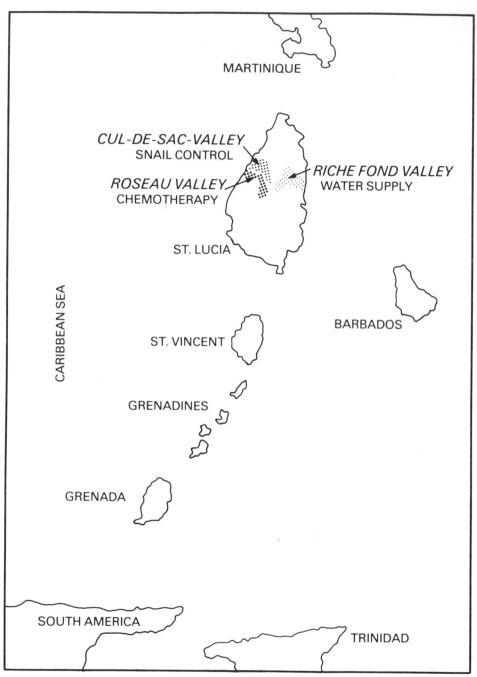

MARTINIQUE

CUL-DE-SAC-VALLEY
SNAIL CONTROL

RICHE FOND VALLEY
WATER SUPPLY

ROSEAU VALLEY
CHEMOTHERAPY

ST. LUCIA

CARIBBEAN SEA

BARBADOS

ST. VINCENT

GRENADINES

GRENADA

SOUTH AMERICA

TRINIDAD

Three separate valleys on the island of St. Lucia in the Caribbean were chosen for the experiment.

do. A banana plant that produces fruit within nine months is a valuable cash crop for anyone who cares to try. Nevertheless the economy of the island is horribly fragile, dependent almost solely on bananas and tourism. The winds of a hurricane or a political crisis can destroy both.

The racial and ethnic origins of the St. Lucians are mixed, and this, too, bears on schistosomiasis. The Arawaks from South America were among the earliest people to arrive and gradually spread northward through all the islands of the Caribbean. Another human tide came in with the Carib Indians, who killed off the Arawak men and married their women. In the sixteenth century first Spanish, then English, privateers dropped in, sometimes by design, sometimes blown off course. The first attempts at colonization by four hundred men from Bermuda and St. Kitts lasted a mere eighteen months, ending in a massacre by the local Caribs. The French arrived in the midseventeenth century, and during the next one hundred fifty years the island changed hands between them and the British fourteen times. The fort on top of the Morne, a hill outside Castries, that rises one thousand feet, became the focus of these struggles. The British finally built a barracks up there that dominated the capital and the harbor approaches. When the island was secure, the Cable and Wireless Company built at the very top of the Morne another barracks whose architecture reflects wealth and confidence. The rooms of the rectangular buildings have most gracious dimensions, with high ceilings; the ground-floor rooms all open onto terraces; the second floor rooms onto balconies that encircle the buildings.

Though the island achieved independence in 1976, the names of parishes, the families, and the plantations still mirror the variety of its settlers. And although it can never be definitely proved, the arrival of slaves was probably crucial for schistosomiasis. The slaves were imported by both the British via Barbados and the French via Martinique and Guadeloupe, but since their transporters dominated different areas of West Africa, the tribal origins of the black population are extremely varied. Many tribes are represented and these can be traced in the slave registers from the plantations. At least seven African tribes can be identified with certainty. Of these at least two, and probably all seven, are from West Africa, including the Congo, where schistosomiasis infections similar to those in St. Lucia have been known for decades. By the end of the eighteenth century there were nearly seventeen thousand slaves on the island, ruled by twelve hundred whites, while another two thousand people had an indeterminate status.

The first official reports of schistosomiasis occurred much later, in 1925. Near the volcanic springs at Soufrière, at the southern end of the island, is an exquisite mountain pool fed by a waterfall whose sides are curtained by tropical ferns, a seductive temptation on a hot day. Even in the 1920s the island had a tourist industry, albeit a small one, and the sulfur baths, with their supposedly health-giving properties, were a great attraction. Three Britishers vacationing near Soufrière bathed in the hot springs, then cooled off in the pool. All three became ill, with symptoms of lassitude and liver and spleen enlargement. Clinical tests in Barbados confirmed schistosomiasis. If three visitors could pick up the infection that quickly, the number of natives infected must have been considerable. Nevertheless local records of the time show that though schistosomiasis was widely disseminated through the population, its prevalence was low. Then after 1950 the disease dramatically and suddenly increased.

This surge was linked to the changeover from sugar cane to banana cultivation. The drainage ditches that crisscross the plantations provide an ideal breeding ground for the snails. The sugar drains dried in the dry season, but now, in the shade of huge banana leaves, these ditches never dry out completely, and there are six hundred miles of them. Hidden among the weeds, the infected snails have ideal breeding conditions. The plantation laborers too have a far greater chance of encountering the cercariae, because cultivation of the banana crop requires them to walk in the drains much more. Unlike sugar cane, banana plantations must constantly be kept free of weeds and sprayed with insecticide. A vicious circle rapidly built up: the more people who were infected, the greater the number of snails infected; the more snails encountered, the more people infected. By simple compounding, the disease incidence climbed, with rural areas showing the highest rates. As more roads were built, the population carried the disease into areas previously free. By 1960 it was being reported everywhere, and with fresh irrigation schemes planned, the incidence was expected to climb even higher.

Consultants from the United Nations' World Health Organization reported that the problem was bad enough to justify a comprehensive control program. Concern about worldwide schistosomiasis was increasing, and a report submitted to both the Academy of National Sciences in the United States and to the British government urged a comprehensive and detailed study that would compare the three known methods of control. Not only was the disease already endemic in many countries, but its boundaries were spreading alarmingly as new irrigation schemes for agriculture in the newly developing nations, especially those in Africa, were built. Schistosomiasis was seen as *the* major threat to economic programs, and was labeled "a disease of development."

The Rockefeller Foundation began to look for an appropriate site for such an experiment. Reconnaissance trips had already been made to Africa, Brazil, and Puerto Rico when the St. Lucian Minister of Health, Dr. François Hunter, appeared in their offices seeking help for St. Lucia. He was told of the Foundation's interest in a detailed study of schistosomiasis control and immediately issued an invitation for its officers to come and see the prospects for themselves.

Arriving in October 1964, they quickly realized that St. Lucia was ideal. Not only was it small, with a population then of just one hundred thousand, but there was a high prevalence of infection. Most important, its topography provided as ideal a situation as would be possible to find. For the valleys were discrete with individual watersheds, and neither the flora and fauna, nor the water of one merged with that of another. This isolation was mirrored in the communities' lives, for footpaths over the hills were either nonexistent or infrequently used, so there was little social contact. The natural contact with water, too, was right: though the villages varied in size, some having several hundred houses, others only twenty or so, all were within walking distance of a river or stream. The women carried water home often several times a day and would regularly go to the rivers to do the laundry, taking along their small children.

Therefore, in 1965, a memorandum of understanding between the government of St. Lucia and the Rockefeller Foundation was signed. Each side "agreed to cooperate in the study of matters affecting the health of the people of St. Lucia and in seeking and applying measures to control disease and, more specifically, schistosomiasis." The idea was to identify three valleys where the incidence of schistosomiasis was high and, over a period of years, systematically apply one of the three known control methods. Then the effects, benefits, advantages, disadvantages, and the costs would all be assessed.

There clearly were three possible ways to achieve control, and success would come not just when people were cured, but only when the chain of infection was irrevocably broken. Two strategies were directed at those vulnerable stages in the parasite's life-cycle while the third was to remove people from the source of infection. One could attack the parasite, either by killing the snails with chemicals thrown into the streams, or by administering worm-killing drugs to infected people. Most difficult of all, one could endeavor to break the habits of generations and wean people away from the rivers. For this though, neither edict, precept, example, nor education alone would be effective. To wean people from their traditional water supplies meant offering reasonable alternatives.

The scientists did have some experience to draw on, for control schemes had been started — and abandoned — in other parts of the world. Most had used single control methods only. Of the various chemicals that killed snails, some were ineffective and some not, but all were very expensive. In Japan and notably in China, control was achieved simply by denying the snail its habitat: swamps were drained and filled. In China the water in irrigation canals was lowered, the muddy banks piled into the center of the channels and the snails buried. Then the banks were lined with concrete, or streams were drained and concrete irrigation pipes laid. At this time snail control alone was the favored method, for drugs were toxic and the standard treatment consisted of twelve injections of an antimony-based compound. Horribly corrosive, the drug caused bad burns if dropped on the skin and since a patient would have to return for twelve consecutive days — an impossible prospect for a subsistence farmer — it was hopeless as a means of mass control. Since water supplies and sanitation, if installed at all, were never put in for schistosomiasis control alone, many scientists erroneously concluded that their impact on the disease would be minimal.

Thus the St. Lucian experiment would be a pioneering undertaking and teams of quite different kinds of scientists were chosen. Where snail control would be tried, biologists would be needed to discover the full details of the snail's life-cycle and when in the year its numbers were greatest, and where most were found. And if the other life in the streams was to be preserved, the animals' ecologic requirements would need to be understood in the finest detail, as would those factors that increased or diminished its population.

The clinicians responsible for chemotherapy would be testing drugs to learn which were most effective, and how and when they were best administered. Should everyone be treated, and how did one find the people with heavy infections? Besides the skills of a clinician and epidemiologist, people with pharmaceutical training had to be recruited, and technical assistants too, trained in tests that ranged from measuring egg counts in people's excreta to others who assisted clinical diagnosis.

Since in the third valley the chosen control method would depend on fresh water supplies and decent sanitation, the skills of the hydraulic engineer would be required, and those of anthropologists, who could investigate the cultural patterns of water use to find out who was going into the streams most frequently, and when and why?

Thus the experiment was initiated. Both the capital costs for the next sixteen years and most of the recurrent ones – nearly $9 million – were met by the Rockefeller Foundation. Other funds came from the Medical Research Council of the United Kingdom, while the government of St. Lucia contributed land for homes and laboratories. The first laboratory was in the old Cable and Wireless barracks on top of the Morne; besides work space, the buildings provided accommodation for visiting researchers and a hospital. Prefabricated buildings were later erected for more laboratories and offices and, in October 1968, the first patient was admitted – the first of four thousand who would ultimately pass through the hospital.

Although several of the staff came from Great Britain, the United States, Australia, Guyana, and several African nations, the majority were St. Lucians. Many had never tackled such jobs before, but they would be trained as scientists and technicians, whether in laboratories, hospitals, or in the field. They would be secretaries or take jobs in the storerooms, or gardens, or in security, and they would provide crucial liaison with the local population. By 1967, when all the teams were operating, some ninety people were involved full time, supplemented by one hundred local health workers and a variety of visiting specialists. The work had to be organized and orchestrated. The person chosen to direct the entire project was Dr. Peter (Pip) Jordan.

Pip Jordan is big and burly and still muscular after a thirty-three-year career in tropical medicine. Over six feet tall, with round, warm, and sometimes very red face, he exudes a feeling of immense strength and capacity. He could have stepped out of a former era (in some ways he did), and like the St. Lucians in the police or customs, wore the old colonial uniform: neat starched shorts and knee-length socks, with the tops turned down in impeccable tidiness.

He graduated with an M.D. from St. Bartholomew's Hospital, London, and after a three-year period in the Royal Navy, returned to study at the London School of Hygiene and Tropical Medicine. There an advertisement in the *British Medical Journal* caught his eye: a scientist was needed to start a research institute in Tanganyika (now Tanzania). He stayed there for over fifteen years, working on another severe tropical parasitic infection, filariasis, and one hot afternoon, on the shores of Lake Victoria in Kenya, he and his wife Jessie, picnicking with their small daughter, Mary, cooled off in the waters. A few weeks later the unmistakable signs of lassitude and general feeling of discomfort appeared: both had contracted schistosomiasis and underwent the full course of twelve agonizing antimony injections.

In 1965 he was offered the job as director of the St. Lucia control project. After several visits to the island he accepted, only after assurances that everyone realized that such a project could never be completed during its first term, five years. He began recruiting staff: Bob Sturrock, British, came at the beginning of the experiment as principal biologist and stayed till 1973, to be replaced by Guy Barnish, also British. So too was Mike Prentice, who had known Jordan in East Africa and had twenty years' experience in Uganda as a field biologist. Joe Cook, American, had attended the Harvard School of Public Health, having become interested in working in international health after training in internal medicine. By chance he met an officer of the Rockefeller Foundation, heard of the St. Lucia project, came down to the island and left eight years later, but only because his two young daughters were then ready for high school education. Gladwin ("Speed") Unrau, American, was raised on a Kansas farm and went to engineering school. He started his career as "sanitary" engineer (the term "environmental" is now substituted). Unrau, who had worked on one schistosomiasis control program in Puerto Rico and another in Egypt, joined the St. Lucia project in June 1965. Peter Dalton, Australian, aptly nicknamed Peter Pumpkin, was an anthropologist with a Ph.D. from the University of the West Indies who just turned up one day off a ship in Castries harbor. Frank Morrison, American, a tough, versatile, down-easter from Maine, was responsible for a battery of vital functions in administration, logistics, mechanical maintenance, and general organization. Fitzroy Henry, Guyanese, was a specialist in health matters, who came to study the wider benefits of water supplies.

So houses were built or rented for wives and families; children were brought over or placed in schools at their home; equipment was ordered and transported; personnel hired and trained; the barriers of paper, customs, and bureaucracy, circumvented, surmounted, or dismantled; and the activity gathered momentum.

Three phases were planned. During the first, from 1971 to 1973, similar information about schistosomiasis would be collected from all three valleys. In the next phase, 1973 to 1976, intensive control methods would be systematically, but separately, applied and their effects evaluated. This phase called for most careful organization, for it was vital that all control work be started at the same time in each valley; otherwise the results would have little validity. The third and final phase, which it was hoped would break the infectious cycle once and for all, would last four years (1976 – 1980). Finally, during 1980 and 1981, the operation would be wound down to levels that could be sustained by the St. Lucian government.

Pip Jordan realized that the people of St. Lucia were really the most important group of all. His scientists' questions might be finely articulated and their experimental methods exquisitely sophisticated, but they were not dealing with planets in the sky or mice in a cage. Nothing could be taken for granted and they would have to understand these people and elicit their cooperation. Only in the valley where snail control was the method would the impact on human beings be negligible. But in the valley where chemotherapy was applied sustained cooperation would be needed, and in the valley where water would be installed, a major change was to be made in long-established patterns of human lives, calling for a social intervention on an unprecedented scale.

Many factors contributed to the personal and communal character of the people. Poverty has driven many to emigrate; 2 percent of the population left in the 1960s and unfortunately the emigrants, primarily male, were generally the better educated and younger (15–45) age group. During the same time the birthrate increased 1.5 percent and the women, who had to work, left their infants in the care of grandmothers or neighbors.

Few St. Lucians own their own land now or ever did. This fact, combined with the vestigial memories of colonialism and the emigration of a crucial segment of the population, makes for a special mix in the rural settlements. Although the four urban areas do have some community focus, village settlements do not. There is neither "village hall," nor square, nor fountain, only one or two rum shops. When Peter Dalton, the anthropologist, asked if he might meet the village mayor or leader he was told that no such person existed. He wrote of the veiled, threatening air overhanging many settlements – a peculiar atmosphere of indolence tinged with violence, especially when neighbors become embroiled in arguments that often end in fisticuffs, or, on occasion, a machete attack.

It was the energy, muscle power, cooperation, and social cohesion of these rural people that the project would need. But attitudes run deep in permanent poverty, so the predominant feeling was mistrust – of all governments, of everyone's motives, and anyone's promises. The people had lived with schistosomiasis for years, so when, one Sunday in April 1967, Erroll Auguste, a government health inspector, spoke from a church pulpit and said that schistosomiasis was a major health problem, it made little stir. When he added that the government was going to do something about it, the unanimous reaction was skepticism. But when suddenly teams of energetic outsiders invaded their valleys, things started to hum.

The three chosen valleys — Cul-de-Sac, Marquis, Richefond — are all comparatively close to Castries. Cul-de-Sac valley was the domain of the biologists whose goal was to shatter the population of the one species of snail, of many on St. Lucia, that harbored the parasite. Marquis valley belonged to the clinicians, who, by killing the parasite in humans, hoped to reduce the number of eggs that would be passed back into the water. In Richefond valley the engineers were going to break contact with the parasite absolutely by providing fresh water. If all the scientists achieved their objectives, then transmission of the disease would be totally broken. So from their commanding position high on the Morne, each team set forth to conquer a different enemy.

Cul-de-Sac valley begins where, after crossing the Morne, the main road drops abruptly to sea level and then turns east and runs right through an enormous banana plantation crisscrossed by irrigation drains. On the fringes of the valley, where the plantation finishes, the road rises along a narrower, steeper section through the few settlements. Here the wooden houses supported above the mud on short stilts punctuate the landscape and here, off the main road, narrow footpaths skirt the ponds and marshes.

Bob Sturrock was the principal biologist until the end of the first phase in 1973, and like Guy Barnish, his successor, was a laboratory biologist. Mike Prentice was the field biologist and together their first task was to find out those techniques that would best eliminate the tiny, smooth-shelled *Biomphalaria glabata*. Actually, so they told me, their very first task was to explode a myth — that the three valleys chosen in St. Lucia were identical. Certainly the human populations might look the same and their incidence of schistosomiasis more or less equivalent, but there the similarities abruptly ended.

To understand the patterns of the snail populations, the biologists had to discover where in the valley they occurred, in what numbers, and whether they were healthy or infected and thus sick. Did most live in the marshes, or in the streams, or in the banana drains? At what time of year were they infected by the parasite, and was this influenced by the rainfall or the movements and numbers of people? Did the numbers of infected snails fluctuate throughout the myriad of habitats? When did the snail shed its cercariae: every minute of the day or only sometimes? Such questions had to be answered before one could even start to kill the animals. And the same information would have to be gathered in the other valleys too in order to answer the main question: Just how and when did people meet up with the snails?

During the first three years the biologists operated on a two-week schedule: flat out in Cul-de-Sac valley during week 1 and in selected habitats in other valleys during week 2. Twenty-six sites in Cul-de-Sac valley, representing all types of habitats – ponds, streams, marshes, banana drains – were regularly sampled and the number of snails counted. In key sites on ponds and streams, one man using a standard scoop would search a fixed area of bank for a given number of minutes. Eight separate stations were also marked out in the marshes and the mud from a three-foot-square area would regularly be scooped unless the marsh was dry, in which case the snails were collected by hand. At the four stations in the banana drains, an iron core was hammered into the mud; back in the laboratory the snails were washed out of the mud extracted by the core.

The technique that showed when the snails shed the cercariae simply involved exposing test tubes of captured snails to the sunlight for one hour. The one used to detect density of the cercariae involved placing mice in the water, supported by a "lifebelt," a cork with a hole in it. There the mouse would sit for a couple of hours around noon, floating with its head above the water, to be examined in the laboratory for infection later. This technique was both expensive and ineffective: in 1969, 9,000 mice were exposed in this way and though 7,594 survived immersion, only twelve infections were found though $10,000 had been spent in maintaining the colony. So another technique was devised which was so successful that it was later adopted in many other worldwide programs. The technique, "sentinel snails," was extremely simple: a simple fiberglass envelope of mosquito netting, stiffened by a plastic rod along two sides and one end, formed the cages. The cages containing healthy, laboratory-bred, snails were placed in the water at the edges of the key sites for twenty-four hours. Once back in the laboratory, the snails were kept for a further twelve days before being crushed and examined for infection.

Things were going along splendidly for the biologists when disaster struck. In the summer of 1970 a heavy tropical storm skirted the island, with winds of hurricane force. Within hours the rivers rose several feet and limpid streams became fast-moving torrents. Trees fell and debris blocked the roads, jammed the culverts, and dammed the streams as ponds and marshes overflowed. The banana drains were clogged as the trees smashed down. In less than twenty-four hours the snails had completely vanished. Overnight all the carefully plotted areas were washed away. It was a shattering blow for the researchers, who had been so precise, so careful, and so hard-working, and they were as depressed as only a scientist can be when the fruits of a carefully contrived experiment are lost, whether by a smashed culture dish on the laboratory floor or failure in a power circuit that turns off an incubator. With his usual buoyancy Pip Jordan encouraged them to look on the bright side and turn the disaster to their advantage. As it turned out, the experience yielded one important lesson that, while humbling, was vital to the success of the control methods they finally devised. The same lesson would be reinforced three years later in 1974, when Hurricane Beulah smashed across the island.

The biologists had initially believed that wiping out the snails would be easy and that, once it was done, the populations might take months to recover. But studies following the storm and the hurricane showed how rapidly the snails could recover from a natural disaster that smashed their habitats and destroyed their population, a situation analogous to destruction by wholesale treatment with chemicals. What was unexpected and worrying was the speed with which the snail population recovered. The critical snail on St. Lucia is hermaphrodite, both male and female, and it regenerated its numbers in just three months flat. This meant that a one-shot mollusciciding job, with effects that woud last forever, was out of the question.

As the snail populations recovered, so too did the scientists' buoyancy, for their studies were turning up a number of highly significant facts. Mad dogs and Englishmen are not the only living creatures that come out in the midday sun: the shedding of the cercariae is triggered by sunlight, so the chances of being infected at dawn are significantly lower than at noon, when the sun is overhead, and the shedding peaks. They learned that differing weather patterns from one year to the next were eventually mirrored in snail population, and though these built up in both still water and streams, the populations in each reached their peak at different seasons and for different reasons. In the rainy season of the summer months, the river snails were washed out by the floods and could not establish colonies, while those in the banana drains, ponds, and marshes still flourished. But when, in the dry winter, these too dried up, the few snails that somehow survived eventually trickled down into the rivers. Here, as the vegetation recovered with the first rains of spring, they quickly reestablished themselves. Though the standing water of ponds and marshes joins with the flowing streams to form the watershed, in them are *two quite separate* snail populations, interlocked in cycles of growth. But of the two populations, it was the one in standing water that was crucial, for it formed the reservoir that constantly replenished the snail population in the streams.

Perhaps then, the scientists reasoned, they should concentrate on the standing water and treat only the snail populations in the marshes, ponds, and banana drains. For if these could be eliminated immediately after the floods, there would be no chance that the snail population in the rivers could be restored. But these habitats were appallingly difficult to treat. In the high marshes, where the vegetation was particularly dense, liquid spray did not always reach the water where snails lay. Dry granules of chemicals were more effective, but so thick was the overgrowth that they did not really penetrate even when sprayed from the air. In one particular marsh at the mouth of Cul-de-Sac valley, the vegetation was so dense that it would have taken six weeks to spray by hand, and since, in the marshes, the number of infected snails was always very low, this would make little impact on the disease. Once again the biologists were driven back to the obvious fact: the standing water of marshes and ponds might be the source that replenished the river snails after the floods but this source was *not* a critical source for transmission of the disease.

When these biological results were laid alongside Dr. Peter Dalton's anthropologic ones, many other important facts came to light. The peak time for shedding of the cercariae – midday – was, unfortunately,   /
also the favorite time for women and children to go down to the river. There was only occasional contamination from humans' excreta in the marshes and the ponds and, surprisingly, it was equally sporadic in the banana drains. A laborer might once defecate in the six hundred miles of banana drain, but the chances of his doing it again in the identical spot were small. So though the standing water in ponds, drains, and marshes was the source of *all* the snail populations; paradoxically, infected snails were rarely found there.

It was quite a different story in the rivers and the streams, however, where repeated human contact provoked repeated contamination. Once the snails had reestablished themselves after the dry season, many became infected, to release thousands more cercariae into the water that infected humans all over again. Here the scientists consistently found many infected snails, and, they decided, it was these they must eliminate.

Given all these facts, logic suggested that the best tactic would be to treat every stream on the island. They tried it once in Cul-de-Sac alone and it took ten weeks. The technique was expensive besides and did great ecologic damage; even if time hadn't been an overriding consideration, futility was. For though the onset of those rains that revived the snail population could be predicted roughly, as could the amount of rain that would fall in so many weeks, in reality no one could say *just* when the ponds would fill or the rivers flood. As Bob Sturrock was later to explain: "The dry season is only about six to eight weeks and given that you can't predict either when it will start, or end, and that it takes ten weeks to spray the whole valley, the chances of missing key sites at critical times when the population is building up again were very high."

The people in the valley were delighted with all the activity in their midst, for though the molluscicide was deadly to aquatic life it was harmless to humans. All along the valley's length people were scooping up hundreds of dying fish and eating them. The biologists were of course concerned about the effects on the flora and fauna in Cul-de-Sac, but in the early years believed it was more important to stop transmission in infected water than to preserve other life.

In 1970, the year they started to implement control, the biologists' grip upon the snail population tightened. They chose first to blanket the snail populations with treatment, then began regular reexamination of the key sites where humans and snails met. By now these index sites had been observed for three years. Infected snails were regularly found there but only there. If schistosomiasis was going to be passed to people it would occur at these points. The biologists certainly would have liked to reduce the snail populations in the standing water too, but as a permanent public health measure, this was totally unrealistic. Many people would be needed and the organized management that the biologists provided during the experiment was far in excess of what any public health authority on a poor island could ever provide. On one occasion, for example, three Ph.D.'s walked ahead of the spray men and, with machetes, cleared the banana trees from the drains after Hurricane Beulah had blown half of them over. There was no way such a degree of manpower or commitment would be available in the future.

In any case other changes were taking place that affected the situation. Geest Industries, the principal landowners in St. Lucia, were abandoning some banana fields because they were uneconomic: they couldn't get enough laborers, for the tourist industry was soaking up the people as waiters or taxi drivers. A banana field is comparatively easy to treat with molluscicide if it is well kept; but if it is neglected and overgrown, it is virtually impossible to get in the molluscicide. Yet such fields, though not transmission points of infection, were still a potential reservoir of snails.

In the light of these changes, and based on their experience of the first three years, Pip Jordan now asked his biologists to draw up a *realistic* public health approach to the control of schistosomiasis in Cul-de-Sac valley for if their methods were to be of any use in other countries, they had to be practical as well as effective. The final strategy recommended concentrated on a routine examination of certain selected sites only. By now the scientists knew a great deal about Cul-de-Sac valley and where these critical sites were. Instead of having to worry about nineteen miles of stream, the biologists knew that only five miles had to be carefully examined. Even within this stretch only a small number of places had to be covered with high surveillance – the actual points where the parasite passed from snails to people. All snails farther away could be ignored.

In 1970 they applied a second blanket treatment throughout the valley, and from then on it was merely a question of routine, monitoring the key sites and applying chemicals when necessary. The routine had to be unrelenting nonetheless. Then for the next five years the compound, bayluscide, was selectively sprayed on the waters of Cul-de-Sac valley, with one further subtle difference: it was sprayed only if, in their monthly searches, the scientists actually found *infected* snails.

Once such control had begun, sentinel snails were again put in the streams to measure infection, and the biologists also continued counting snails at the places where before they had found many infected. They still found snails all right, but now only a few had the parasite. So long as human beings continued to come back to the rivers, there would be some infection, even if the snail population was drastically reduced in number. The biologists could halt transmission of schistosomiasis temporarily, but while the people remained untreated they would pass eggs into the water. The study in Cul-de-Sac finally concluded that, <u>even after two years of mollusciciding, a</u> constant pool of infection came in from people. Still it was clear that the people of Cul-de-Sac were far less affected by the disease, however, because some transmission of infection was being stopped.

Quantitatively the figures were these: during the control period the infection rate in all children, aged ten and under, dropped from 22 to 4 percent; the infection rate in the sentinel snails also dropped from 3.9 to 1.1 percent during the same four years. This led to a gradual dying off of the schistosome worms, which in turn led to a fall in the prevalence of the disease in people of all ages. By 1975, when the intensive control phase ended, transmission of infection was virtually nonexistent in the whole of Cul-de-Sac. By then the clinicians were screening the people too, and anyone still excreting eggs was treated with drugs. During the last maintenance phase, spraying of the streams continued on a monthly basis in Cul-de-Sac valley, but in the new, subtle way, focused only on those river areas where people lived or areas used for routine sanitary purposes (laundry, bathing, excretion). This technique proved just as effective as widespread spraying and, of course, considerably less expensive. By 1980, the last full year of the program, when seven hundred children in Cul-de-Sac valley were examined, only *two* were found to be carrying eggs. This was magnificent success.

Yet in some measure the biologists' tactical conclusions were ironic. When the program started, snail control was considered best; when it ended they knew that mollusciciding alone could never get rid of schistosomiasis. In the 1960s people had talked about eradicating the snails; in the 1980s they no longer did, for they knew by then that snails are adapted to recover their numbers very rapidly after disasters. They talk now only of "managing" the snail populations, and no one imagines that schistosomiasis can be controlled by attention to the secondary host alone.

Dr. Joe Cook's target was the worm inside the man; his main locations were the Victoria Hospital in Castries, the clinical wards and the small hospital on top of the Morne, and Marquis valley with its main health center at Babboneau. Marquis valley is situated in the center of the island, on the fringe of the northern quarter. Each day Dr. Cook had merely to drive a few miles west from the Morne, along a dirt road that traversed a ridge, with stunning views over Castries and the northern, driest section of St. Lucia. The red clay road winds along the ridge and down the valleys before climbing again through the ten settlements of the Marquis valley. Small wooden shacks above the mud, and a few concrete houses, are flanked by the odd patch of land where the people grow vegetables. All the time a warm steam rises from the earth as the sun burns off the last shower.

Joe Cook's first task during the first phase was to organize baseline clinical studies in all three valleys. Then in Marquis valley alone he would begin a control program of drug therapy and would also treat patients from all over the island. Four thousand people would pass through his wards on the top of the Morne. Here his team tested all the new drugs that were coming in and did clinical investigations into the severe cases of schistosomiasis.

Though one essential procedure was simple, compliance was not easy, for the clinical team needed a stool specimen from *everyone* in the valleys. These were obtained through a health education unit, led by Erroll Auguste, that covered the whole island. Although Auguste knew he couldn't meet every inhabitant, he took his unit to every settlement. So in the discotheques and the movie houses of the towns, during the intermission between a romantic film and a cartoon, Auguste would give a short talk on the parasite and what should be done to avoid it, and what the control program offered. He could reach nearly one thousand people, of all ages, at just one movie house. Those more religiously inclined – Roman Catholics, Baptists, or Seventh Day Adventists – would hear his talk between the collection and the sermon, for the educators were given pulpit time during Mass in Castries Cathedral as well as during church services all over the island. As the months passed Auguste took along people who had once had the disease but who were now cured. His group also monitored the streams, chasing away the mothers and the children from them. Going from house to house, he explained why fecal specimens were needed and how "poop," as the people called it, would be collected and every member of the family must give a specimen. He would return with the results and would explain to anyone infected just what the doctors would do to rid the belly of worms. Getting the specimens once was easy; getting them for a second, a third, and a fourth time was considerably more difficult. Unless they were seriously ill, men would give a sample once but never again.

Everyone in the Marquis valley lived within three kilometers of the Babboneau Health Centre, and ninety percent of the people in the valley gave the first stool specimen. Notices were delivered door to door by the team of health aides saying when people could come in for screening, and those infected for treatment. Though there was no compulsion, the teams went through every village methodically, offering therapy wherever infection was found. If people missed treatment, the health workers returned again and again till they found them. The notices were sent out one day before the clinic so there was no time for people to forget, and though not all could read, enough did. Others would take the notice to a neighbor. Then the teams fanned out once more to seek cooperation from those they had missed.

Once again, after three years, the intensive control phase started and 1,042 people excreting worm eggs were treated in Marquis. Many houses had radios and since St. Lucia's most popular disc jockey was a well-known health buff, Joe Cook could stroll into the national radio station and get free air time whenever he liked. The public announcement broadcast called the residents of Babboneau to attention and said which three days in the week treatment for bilharzia would be given. It finished with the clarion call, "You are encouraged to come at your appointed time.

If everyone cooperates in this campaign, we can get rid of the bilharzia worm in the Marquis valley."

The first treatments were two intramuscular injections of hycanthone, though a few very young children were given niridazole. There were daily follow-ups on all patients receiving hycanthone, for the drug can have side effects, varying from vomiting to jaundice, though these never occurred in St. Lucia. Two health aides would make the house calls and if any member of the household was away, they would return over and again rather than ask patients to make a special journey to the health center. When the program was in full spate, Joe Cook had fourteen such nurse aides working with him; afterward many went on to more important jobs in the health service. Then, in 1975, a new drug, oxamniquine, was introduced which could be given by mouth in a single dose and which had fewer side effects. This was to have a dramatic effect not only in St. Lucia but all over the world, for it and praziquantel, another anti-bilharzia drug, are a clinician's dream.

Oxamniquine was developed by the Pfizer Group in the United Kingdom and ultimately would receive the Queen's Award for exports. The drug emerged from two research strategies: one looked at the biochemistry of the worm's metabolism and tried to block the pathways; the other screened other drugs in existence since the 1930s, to see if they were any use. It took three years for the chemists to do the screening tests in laboratory animals that established the best dosages, the pharmaceutical properties, and the toxicology data. Then there was the usual clinical trial, during which oxamniquine was found to be wonderfully effective, though only against the form of schistosomiasis found in Africa and Latin America. As a bonus, not only did the drug prove safe but, better still, it was just as effective when given by mouth as by needle.

The switch to oxamniquine coincided with the arrival of a new staff member, Dr. Ed Cooper, from the Children's Hospital in Washington, D.C. He would stay to monitor the permanent control program that would be set up when the experiment finished. Once the switch was made to a single-dose oral drug with few side effects, follow-up visits to drug recipients were unnecessary. Nevertheless the health aides still made regular house calls throughout all the four years' control, on all 1,042 patients. And though the side effects were minimal, nevertheless, as Joe Cook emphasized, patients were carefully monitored especially if they had had any illness in the past.

Since oxamniquine was still in its developmental stage, there were serious discussions in New York and St. Lucia thrashing out the

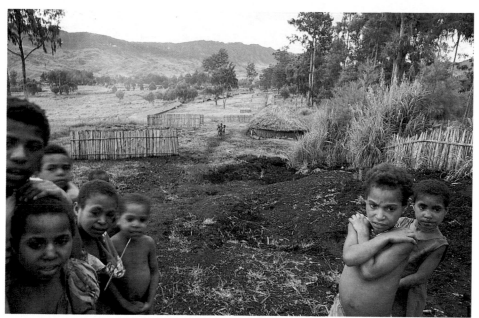

Gajdusek discovered that kuru victims were predominantly women and children. (Compix)

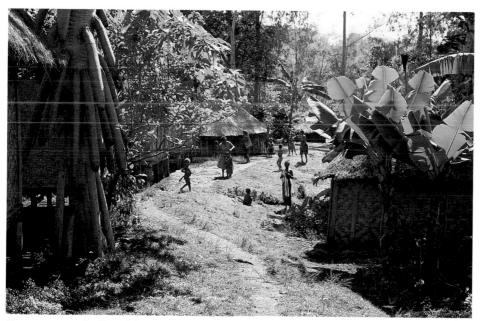

Every aspect of village life was checked and rechecked in the search for clues. (Axel Poignant)

Quest for the Killers

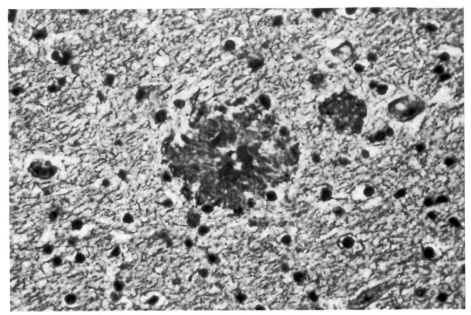

The "kuru" plaque–as seen under the microscope. (Michael Johnstone)

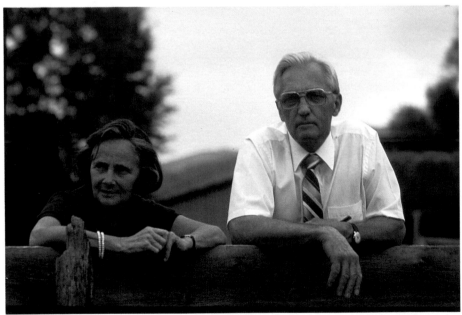

June Goodfield with Dr. Bill Hadlow. (Michael Johnstone)

Quest for the Killers

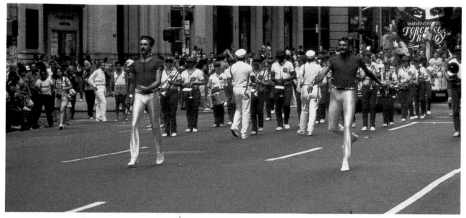

Gay Day parade in New York. (Michael Johnstone)

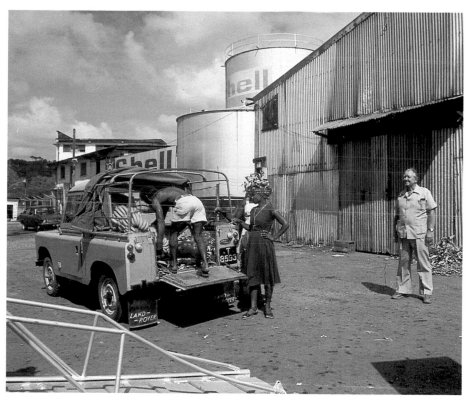

Pip Jordan waits at Castries Harbour for Mike Prentice. (Michael Houldey)

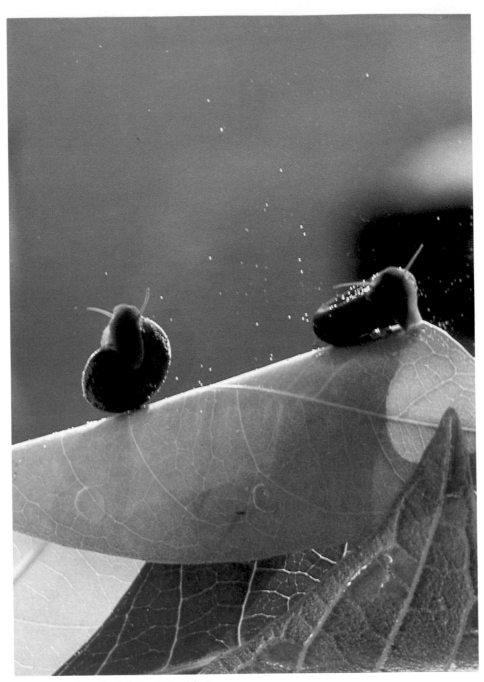

The cause of it all. (Michael Houldey)

Quest for the Killers

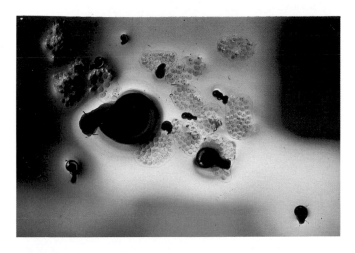

A. *The snails shed their eggs into the water.*

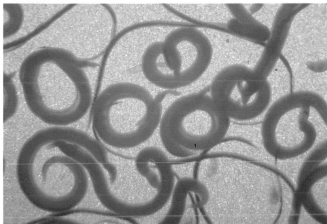

B. *Adult parasitic worms.*

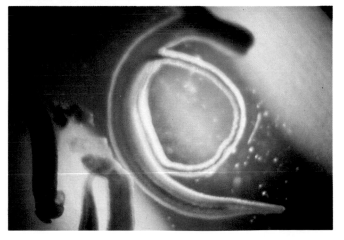

C. *The male and female worms join together.*

Quest for the Killers

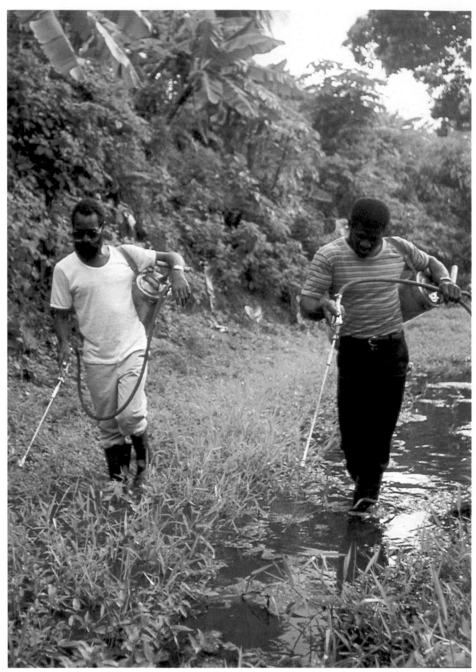

Julian Alexander and Anthony Callender spray the streams. (Michael Houldey)

Quest for the Killers

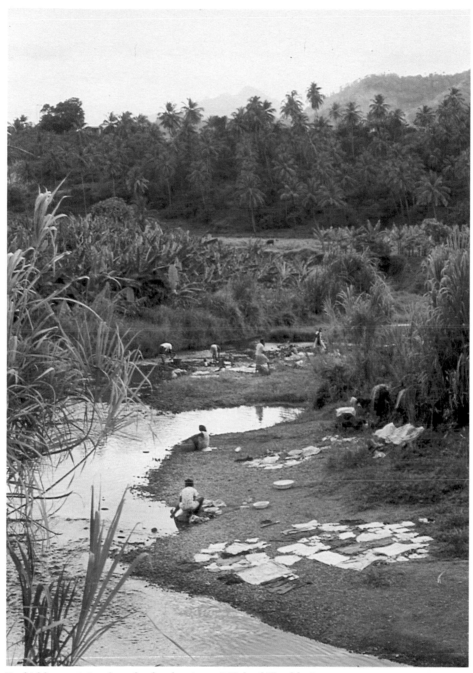

Forbidden activity: laundry by the river. (Michael Houldey)

Quest for the Killers

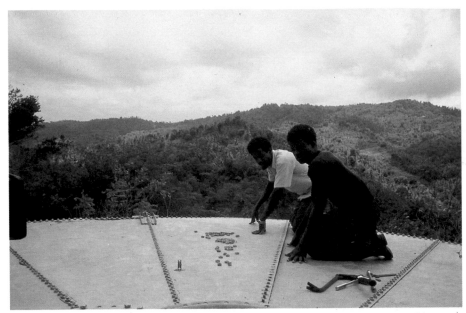

Water tank at the very top of the jungle slope above the villages. (Michael Houldey)

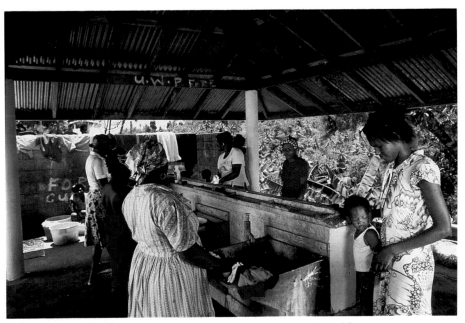

The community laundry was built for the women. (Michael Houldey)

Quest for the Killers

matter of informed consent. The protocols planned were not totally experimental, for the drugs were being used in London and the Commonwealth countries, having been cleared by the World Health Organization and the Dunlop Committee for Drug Safety in the United Kingdom. (St. Lucia was still an associated state of the British Commonwealth.) But since the first one, hycanthone, was not without complications Pip Jordan and Joe Cook discussed the issue at length with the St. Lucian government and it was at the government's request that the consent form usual in Western hospitals was not presented. St. Lucian officials argued that the people would find the need for consent confusing.

Treatment was not confined to patients in Marquis valley, though. Patients were referred from all over the island and a large number came from a small town, Denier, which spreads over a glorious area of rocks, sandy beaches, and trees, along the Atlantic side. Denier had a high incidence of disease and lay in the catchment area of the Richefond valley, where water supplies were the control method. Among the patients who came to Joe Cook was a family of fourteen whose children had such severe disease that their livers and spleen were badly impaired. He treated them all, but one day the four-year-old girl and the six-year-old boy were brought in to him very sick. The girl was started on treatment straight away but the boy had a high fever.

"I felt at the time it was schisto," said Joe Cook.

I still . . . I will never know. I couldn't treat him right away because of the fever, for I had to see what else might be going on and I certainly didn't want to give him any complex compounds while in that condition. But I was called out in the night. He'd had a seizure and by the time I got to the hospital he was dead. I had to do the autopsy and I am not a pathologist. We sent sections off to Alan Cheever in America, one of the most preeminent schistopathologists in the whole world, and he said that this infection was as bad as any he had ever seen. Well, that was quite unusual for St. Lucia, where we rarely saw the problem to this extent. But this sort of thing sticks in your mind for a long time, for who knows? If he had received treatment a little earlier it might have made a difference, but on the other hand it might not. We don't know. I treated the whole family in the end. His sister had an enormous liver, but now she is very well. I have still got pictures of them around me.

This experience was indeed strikingly rare: four thousand patients with advanced schistosomiasis were successfully treated and by 1978 the hospital on the top of the Morne was closed. There were no more patients to admit.

The clinicians' success in reducing infection in their valley was as dramatic as the biologists'. Their studies had shown that settlements up the hill in Marquis had lower rates of schistosomiasis than those on the valley floor, where the dasheen marshes, the small plantations, and the rivers provided better habitats for the snails than the fast streams of the slopes. In these valley settlements though, the incidence in children one to ten years fell from 23 to 2.5 percent and even higher up the hills it fell from 6 to 3 percent. But it was far easier to get a rapid reduction when the infection rates were initially high than it was to get an already low rate down even lower. The last egg, or parasite, or snail, is always the most difficult to eliminate, and in Marquis valley infection was permanently sustained by a small core of people who consistently refused treatment.

The dramatic success of the chemotherapy on the human population had its impact on the snail population of Marquis valley and mirrored the success of Cul-de-Sac. Though sentinel snails during the two years before the control began were infected at the usual rate, once the human population had been treated, not one infected animal was ever seen again, though over five thousand were examined. However, during the last four years of the project, transmission of schistosomiasis started climbing again in two of nine Marquis settlements. There could be several reasons, Joe Cook explains. First, only 80 percent of the people in these settlements would take treatment compared to 90 percent in the others. Moreover, although by then community water supplies had been brought in, the people still continued to use rivers as a back-up. Most important, there was an influx of untreated migrant workers returning to the Marquis valley who had been infected in other places.

In certain respects those studying Richefond valley, where fresh water would be the control method, had the most fascinating job. True, they had more headaches and, in sheer physical effort, would have strenuously to exert themselves, and they would be involved in a major tragedy. Yet it was in Richefond that the teams of St. Lucian and foreign field workers, with their promises and projects, came face to face with the quirks and pride of ordinary human beings.

Richefond valley was chosen because it was almost virgin territory so far as water was concerned and because the communities were clustered in small groups that made possible a water distribution scheme that could be easily studied. Some standpipe water had been provided to a number of rural settlements in the island, but too often the water was either inadequate in quantity or the hand pumps delivering it broke down. So the people were still returning to the rivers. By 1966 four thousand people on the north side of the Richefond valley were sharing communal water, but this did little to control schistosomiasis. In the pools that collected at the base of the standpipes, the infected snails established themselves.

To reach Richefond valley meant driving the length of Cul-de-Sac valley, then climbing the foothills the heights of the rain forest, and finally snaking down again round a steep hairpin bend before cutting into the hinterland. When the program started, the roads did not go all the way and the team had a hard thirteen-mile slog there and back every day.

Speed Unrau, who built the Richefond water system, was the very first staff member to arrive, in June 1975, and was also responsible for all the preliminary work on accommodation and the laboratory buildings. While he and his engineering team were planning their scheme, the biologists and clinicians were, once again, doing baseline studies in Richefond valley to draw a picture there, too, of the snail populations and the human infection. If the people's contact with infected water was to be broken, details on the nature of that contact and the occasions that provoked it needed to be ascertained. So while Speed Unrau's engineering team was surveying, Peter Dalton's anthropology team was observing. For 105 days he and his local helpers followed the pattern of people's lives: How often did they go to the rivers and who, and why, and when, and how wet did they actually get? So as to cover all the seasons, these studies spread over fifteen months, their timing adjusted so that each of fifteen sites was observed on each of the seven days per week. Stationed on the banks the anthropologists would record the name, age, and sex of the person at the river, the time they arrived and left, what they did and how much of their body went into the water; they would note the weather conditions and the flow in the river. Some two thousand villagers, from the settlements of Grande Rivière, Grande Ravine, Debonair, Thomazo, and Mor Panache (patois for Montparnasse) were their "laboratory" subjects.

Though it was known that women doing laundry would not undergo total immersion, nevertheless the scientists believed they would be in prolonged contact with the water. But this turned out not to be so. Women were certainly by the river during those dangerous noon hours, when the hundreds of thousands of cercariae were shed, but most of the washing was done on the banks, where the clothes were scrubbed with hard soap, then banged on the rocks. For a short time as hands were immersed to rinse, feet would be in up to the ankles, but that was all. The observation that turned out to be crucial was quite surprising: even more than the laborers who waded in the six hundred miles of banana drains, it was the children who had the greatest contact with water. Taken down to the rivers by their mothers as soon as they could toddle, they would play on the banks and in no time at all would be splashing or swimming, immersed for as many hours as it took the women to finish the washing. Though they went to school when they were five, they would still return to the rivers. They came to help their mothers, to swim, and to catch crayfish. After the spate in the rainy season, when the long, hot humid days of the tropical summer set in, and the heat and the moisture hang so heavy that it is an effort even to raise a hand, the rivers run clear again and the urge to bathe is overwhelming. The waters eddy under the banks and form deep pools that tempt us seductively – and dangerously – as any siren. Consistently exposed from babyhood to adolescence, the children were at the greatest risk. This was the picture from Dalton's studies, and once the water had come to Richefond, he would repeat them.

Unrau's team meanwhile surveyed all the water sources in the valley to find the best to supply. They were anxious to use gravity flow systems, so as to reduce the need for pump maintenance, but the terrain was so rough that, although in a few places they could get to within fifty feet of the summit ridge, they would still have to use pumping equipment. This first survey showed Pip Jordan the difficulties they now faced in engineering and the volume of labor required to dig trenches, lay plastic pipes, build a pumping station, and supply electricity. All the connecting, welding, molding, and tightening would have to be coordinated in one massive effort. And it was essential to bring this scheme in on time, for if the subsequent results were to have any validity, the control phase in Richefond valley *had* to start at the identical moment as in Cul-de-Sac and Marquis.

Pip Jordan called a meeting in the Thomazo rum shop to explain Unrau's plans and get help. In the small, dark room, the scheme was explained to an audience of wary adults and curious children; a St. Lucian, Urban Glace, was introduced as the director and liaison. Pip Jordan was eloquent: the project would, he said, bring them the best water in St. Lucia. But the St. Lucians didn't believe him. Then on Palm Sunday in 1970, Erroll Auguste climbed into the pulpit once more, to announce officially that the water scheme was going ahead. They didn't believe him either. The burden of their total skepticism, combined with the exhausting effort the scheme demanded, weighed heavily on the staff.

They understood why the villagers were caustic and dismissive. For years the government had promised water and nothing had been done.

The teams, the people thought, were just another lot of fancy foreigners who made fine promises that would come to nothing, and who, past experience would suggest, were doing this out of a self-interest not yet clear. Jordan was scrupulously honest though: it would be very hard work, everything having to be done with human muscle power, but it would be done. He wanted to show that such a scheme *could* be built and that people in other developing nations could build similar schemes themselves. He was determined to fulfill his promise to the people of Richefond.

The first water came to Grande Ravine, just one of five settlements in the valley, a village set back from the main road in the interior. About half a mile from the settlement, the track crosses a river where the women went to fetch water, and then climbs steeply, curving sharply right up through the village. The houses are simply strung on either side of the road. The first water Unrau supplied came from shallow marshy ground through which a stream ran, with a constant, strong flow. An infiltration gallery was built in the muddy earth by the stream and nearby was the pumping station that would lift the water into the reservoir tank situated in the middle of Grande Ravine. It seemed an easy job to capture this surface water, for there was plenty of it. In fact the job was appallingly difficult and the work had to be conducted at a furious pace.

From the pumping station one pipe ran out toward the stream; at the end of the pipe three trenches were dug, each fanning out at 120°, and into these trenches perforated pipes were laid. The theory was that the surface water would simply seep through the perforations back into the central pipe, and then to the pumping station where it would be lifted up to the tank. The practical reality was quite another matter, for the team was working through the rainy season and the central collecting chamber collapsed, not once, but over and over again. They would regularly arrive in the morning to find the previous day's labor destroyed. When the chamber was finally finished, they had to work equally fast to concrete it, and then they discovered that there wasn't really enough water, so they had to tap a second stream too. In one day, using manual labor alone, they connected a half mile of pipe, working all through the day and often through the night as well. Once the pumping station was finished, they tapped the electricity to run the engine.

Once it was clear that water would come to Grande Ravine, anthropologist Peter Dalton convened a meeting, in the village rum shop. Twenty-four people from the settlement turned up; only a few were young and there were no women. He explained the strategy of schistosomiasis control once more and the other benefits that household water would bring, then suggested that the residents should each help dig the trenches from the holding tank to their houses. Though the owner of the rum shop also spoke eloquently of the need to support the program, most residents were highly suspicious, not only of both men but of the government, who they said "promise everything, but do nothing." They were equally hostile to the revenue men, who they believed would now make an appearance and tax them heavily for the water. They continued to distrust the apparent lack of guile shown by all those working on the scheme, whether St. Lucians or foreigners. One small rift in the wall of their mistrust appeared when a few villagers pointed out that at least the white men were helping dig the trenches, so were clearly *trying*.

Despite the general lack of enthusiasm it was decided that the next Saturday would be a suitable time to start digging. Thirteen men turned up and the main line was quickly completed. The next Saturday it rained too heavily for work. On the third Saturday only a few men showed, but some small boys tried to help and the trench progressed halfway to its target. The fourth Saturday was the festival of La Margarite and every weekend for the next two months the celebrations continued. Next there was a row between the government and the plantation owner. The government wished to purchase land near the village and provide not only electricity and water but fresh settlers. While this issue was being debated, the pipe laying remained stalled. By the time it finally resumed Speed Unrau had had quite enough and was determined to make a change, one dictated by the total lack of progress. He issued an edict: each household was required to dig that portion of the trench running through their yard. If they did not, water would not be connected to their house.

This had an immediate effect. The trenches were quickly completed, but now the digging was done entirely by the women and children. There were some heated arguments, even blows, between those who had completed their trenches but who still had no water and their neighbors above who had not completed *their* trenches and so were causing the delay. There were disputes too between tenants and landlords about who would pay any costs incurred, even though there were none. But finally the job was done.

Since the supply below the settlement would not be sufficient, Speed Unrau had been forced to turn his attention to the hill above. He decided to capture as his main supply, water from a steep valley a mile away. They would build a dam and place a reservoir tank high on top of the hill. Later Unrau commented, "You know, no one had ever tried this kind of thing on the island before and Pip teased me – actually *accused* me – of selecting the most difficult site of all for the tank. But I showed him over the rest of the valley and he saw that other sites would be even worse. There was no avoiding it: we needed that height in order to get the pressure."

The feat of capturing the water and building the now notorious Thomazo tank on top of the horrendous Thomazo hill involved a near legendary feat that is still recounted in St. Lucia. Laying plastic pipe down from the pumping station to the five villages in the valley, and up to the top of the hill, where the reservoir tank would be situated, were the easiest tasks. The women transported the plastic pipe and the men dug the trenches along a rough stony track, passing first through a banana plantation, then along the side of a hill and, a mile farther, over muddy, sticky soil, to the head of the valley. The sides of the valley were very steep, and large boulders had to be carried away. But yard by yard, slowly hacking away with machetes, they cut through the forest, dug the trenches, and connected the pipeline.

It now takes only a hot half-hour's walk along that path to reach the pumping station that pushes the water up to the Thomazo tank on top of the hill. Here, the area is dark and isolated. The St. Lucians hated the place; they found it spooky. Few people will go to the rivers after dark, Urban Glace told me, but his group had had to spend several nights and weekends working there.

That dam and tank constituted the most difficult water system Speed Unrau would ever build in his career, for the site was uncompromisingly difficult. Though the water was pristine, uncontaminated, and plentiful, the villages where it was to be delivered were on the wrong side of an intervening ridge. Over and over Unrau's team had surveyed the area, desperately whacking their way through jungle, trying to find an easy way to get the water across the ridge while still achieving a head of pressure that could take water to two thousand people in four hundred houses in five villages from the top to the bottom of Richefond.

How do you place a 40,000 gallon tank on the steepest of rocky hills smothered in the thickest of jungles with no path? Many ways were possible, but the engineering team could only seriously consider a few. The obvious solution was a helicopter and one was for hire in Puerto Rico, but this would have cost a hundred thousand dollars and though the program had money, it was not *that* rich. Speed Unrau and Frank Morrison worried for hours and finally figured out another, cheaper, way.

One by one, the tank sections would be pulled up the mountain and assembled in situ on top. The preparation took longest; inch by inch, a trail had to be hacked through the jungle up a 45° slope. At the bottom they built a concrete platform and ramp, and rigged a pulling device, with pulleys, a truck-mounted winch and nine hundred feet of thick nylon rope that Speed Unrau had found in a local store. Since the sled carrying each section uphill was under lethal tension and would catapult upward if it ever became unhooked, the operation was controlled by walkie-talkies. As operators of the base vehicle did the winching, the rest were pushing, shoving, balancing, steering, and ducking, as each section of the tank was maneuvered up the hill. People walked alongside to prevent the sled being jammed and to make sure that the rope ran free. Volunteers were hard to find for such tough work, so people were paid the going rate – 25 cents an hour for men and 19 for women.

There were some frightening moments. "We were hauling up one big twenty-foot pipe," says Unrau, "and several of the fellows let go when they should have been holding on, and Urban Glace got beaned with a swaying pipe. He never became unconscious but we didn't know just how hard he had been hit. We had three people make a three-man hold into a sort of carriage and carted him down the hill on his back. Luckily he wasn't badly hurt."

It took twelve weeks to complete the tank. From pulling, shoving, and straining, they went to welding, fitting, and annealing. Finally in July 1971, the stopcocks opened, the taps were turned on, and four thousand gallons of clean, filtered water were pumped from the dam up into the Thomazo tank to drop to Grande Ravine by gravity. The pump was inspected daily by Urban Glace, who now became the water supervisor for Richefond. Each house had a standpipe in the yard; a single hard push on the plunger released a gallon of water. Though Unrau and his men say that they have never worked harder on any project to meet such a tight schedule, the compensations were tremendous. Unrau reminisces:

I remember one old lady in her eighties. There was the water coming out of her pipe and she just sat down on the floor in her doorway and began to cry. "I never dreamt," she said, "that there would come a time in my lifetime when I would have water in my own yard." There was another lady I was greatly fond of, one of those picturesque rugged individuals, also in her eighties. Her husband was over ninety and they owned a small piece of land. But they gave it to us for one of the public showers – a crude shower sure, but the first – and that meant we had to cut down their banana plants. Well, when the water came in – I don't know if you can imagine a lanky, West Indian lady in her eighties dancing round the tub. But that's what she did. She was so happy, for she had been going better than a mile every day to carry water on her head in order to get it home.

Her delight was widely shared: in one area alone two hundred tons of water had been carried *each day* by the women, an enormous physical effort.

The celebratory parties went on for days and yet, as the vigilant eyes of Peter Dalton's helpers observed, the water might be there but the people were not leaving the river. Their next batch of studies proved crucial, for they highlighted a neglected social factor. One could provide communal standpipes as the government had, or one in every home, as the control program did, yet if the river were not far away people would still return. Not until communal laundries were provided, where the women could chat and the children play just as they had on the river bank, was the chain of habit severed. Doing the laundry was as much a social occasion as a chore.

The communal laundry in Grande Ravine is next to the old reservoir tank and there are many such all over the island. Simple structures, they are a series of six concrete basins attached to a middle spine; each faucet yields water only when pressed, delivering two gallons per shot. Communal concrete shower units, the men's opposite the rum shop and the women's farther below, are similarly designed. A press of the pedal, or the pull of a handle, and a shot of water shoots over the head.

The water was such a success that other villagers began clamoring for standpipes and laundry units. Dalton's studies continued, his people watching at the same places, on the same days, at the same times. Laundry in the river quickly dropped to 60 percent of its former level and swimming to 30 percent. But even this contact was still too great. Now an intensive campaign of health education began and it was this, and the laundry units, that at last weaned the women from the river and the children with them. Small, simple, concrete swimming pools were also built for small children and while these were immensely popular to begin with, they have not been an unqualified success. The water could easily be chlorinated but the people were sometimes reluctant to use them as they equated still water with dirty water. There was also difficulty keeping everything clean. The intentions may have been there, but the humdrum, daily jobs of cleaning, removing leaves, throwing in chlorine, scrubbing, tidying up, marked the point where, in some settlements, the system fell down. Some villages now have their own rotation of women volunteers for the laundry and shower units; others employ someone, paid by a 25 cent to 50 cent

(EET) levy. Yet other villages expect the Ministry of Health not only to keep the system in repair but to clean it too.

Nevertheless, once the entire system was installed, people returned to the river for only two reasons: for toilet purposes, or when the electricity failed and the water stopped, and so far as schistosomiasis was concerned, Richefond now followed the same pattern as had Cul-de-Sac and Marquis. In five years new infections rapidly fell, from 30.6 percent to 12 percent. At this point it stuck, possibly because the valley children went to a school in an area without piped water and were exposed there to fresh infections. In the final phase during 1975 – 1976, when the actual control experiment had ended and drug treatment was given everywhere, the incidence dropped further, down to 6 percent.

To draw truly valid conclusions, the engineers had left six settlements on the northern side of Richefond valley without piped-in water so the rate of infection there could be compared with the rest of the valley. Even though the government quickly provided a few communal standpipes in these six settlements, placed at intervals along the road, the people still used the river, and in the five years of the experiment the prevalence of infection here actually *rose*. So the government scheme, costing eighteen dollars a head to install, did not reduce the transmission of schistosomiasis although the control scheme at twenty-two dollars a head did. Clearly the success of the one scheme could not lie in the magic sum of four dollars. So where did it lie?

The difference depended first on the provision of laundry units that provided a social setting for laundry and on *individual* standpipes in every household's backyard. These factors weaned people from the river and, as Jordan and his colleagues were quick to note, once the capital cost of bringing water to a village has been borne, the extra cost of giving every household its own tap is minimal. This is not only convenient but healthy too, for mud at the base of shared standpipes is easily contaminated and this seems to have been the second factor that accounted for increase in the disease in those six settlements under the government scheme.

Oddly enough the program revealed that one other factor, – the provision of toilets, which, on the face of it, seemed most important for schistosomiasis control, – though influential, was not crucial. Traditionally people had used the rivers or selected points on their land or in the plantations for elimination. Simple latrines had already been installed in St. Lucia and their capital cost met by the Rotary Clubs of America. Basic structures, a plastic pedestal on a concrete slab over a six-foot deep hole, the latrines required only a little water poured in to remain clean. After a time the pit was filled with earth and the structure moved to a new pit. Speed Unrau wanted latrines installed in all three valleys. Plastic ones, designed in Australia and modified for use in Fiji, were tried in St. Lucia. But the curve was all wrong for steep island slopes, so Unrau redesigned them and demonstrated their use with overripe bananas. They didn't really affect the control of the disease, because water to flush them might not be regularly available, and in any case, they could be used at home but not at work in the fields. Once water supplies were installed, however, the population did not *want* to use the rivers for sanitary purposes, certainly not those that were their water source. Thus the more latrines provided, the better.

Nothing whatever was any use at all, the scientists found, without simultaneous programs of health education. So the coup-de-grace against schistosomiasis was delivered in a lively campaign, conducted by M. Celestin, head of the local Borstal, and his assistant, Thomas James. Celestin is a political pamphleteer and parliamentary candidate of the old style, who happily campaigned actively throughout the island. As economic development starts up, health rights become political issues; this is true everywhere in the world. His campaigns reached even into the secondary schools, where solemn teachers in sober dress would deliver the message to solemn children in school uniforms. Soon everyone throughout the entire island knew a great deal about the control of schistosomiasis.

Many people had given sixteen years of their energetic lives to the experiment, but Speed Unrau was to give much more. One day in 1977, he finished work and returned home early. There was a sour-sop tree in Unrau's yard and he noted some particularly fine fruit on the branches, which he thought he would retrieve before the birds. His wife said, "Oh, don't bother; we have plenty," but Speed replied, "well, Urban Glace and the boys are still working and they like sour-sop real well. I'll just pick the fruit and take it out to them in the morning." He climbed to the usual spot, in a tree he'd climbed a hundred times before – and fell only nine feet. A lot of branches crashed down too, which should have cushioned his fall, but from the freak way in which he fell on a boulder, he broke his tenth thoracic vertebra. Now a paraplegic, he lives in Florida, permanently confined to a wheelchair.

Gradually the program moved into the final phase where methods were devised so that in the future, the St. Lucians themselves could control schistosomiasis. People were trained, or retrained, as biological field technicians, or as diagnostic technicians, or as health educators, or hydraulic engineers, by the core of people who had stayed for sixteen years.

But other people too, who made valuable contributions to the pool of knowledge, had come and gone. One such visitor, Mr. Pierre Peters, was in the eyes of St. Lucians a very special visitor, indeed, for the St. Lucians recognized him as one of their own. Now senior technician in the Department of Geographic Medicine at Case Western Reserve University, he has made a vital contribution to schistosomiasis control, and his interest in the disease has taken him back to his "roots" in ways never imagined by Alex Haley.

Among Mr. Peters's ancestors were slaves transported to the New World. His father was chief of the Balunda tribe in the southern part of the Belgian Congo, now Zaire. His mother, the youngest of the chief's four wives, died while giving birth. Tribal custom dictated that the baby be given to the chief's brother since if the other wives mistreated the child, evil spirits from his mother would return to haunt them. But instead of taking the baby home, his uncle ran to a small clearing in the jungle, the haunt of lions and leopards, and there left him, expecting the tiny body to be reduced to a few bones by the next day. Peters never learned why the man returned the following morning, but the day-old baby was still alive. His uncle was terrified: the evil spirits would now surely concentrate on *him*. So he ran several miles to the nearest mission station and there he left the child.

The station was run by two fundamentalist Baptist missionaries from the United States. They adopted the baby, gave him their last name, and baptized him Pierre André, the name of a popular radio announcer in the United States they admired. He lived with them and their two daughters for ten years, but when they were finally transferred home he had to remain behind, for the Belgian authorities refused to let him go. For a further five years he lived with the missionaries who replaced his parents, along with three more adopted children. Eventually the Peters family returned and took the teenage boy to another station in the northern Congo. Here he went to school, but when his two sisters reached high school age the missionaries again had to return to Lancaster, Pennsylvania, and again Pierre André Peters was refused an exit permit.

Now seventeen, he looked around for work and heard about Dr. Major Donald Price from the Walter Reed Army Hospital in Washington, D.C., who was starting a parasitology laboratory in the Congo and needed a translator. Peters got the job. Price's major interest was schistosomiasis and soon the young man was learning about the disease that would preoccupy him for the rest of his life. In 1960 the Congo became independent Zaire, and two days before independence the backlash against the former white overlords erupted. So Major Price flew to Uganda and Peters and a friend followed, riding the one thousand miles on a motorbike.

When, three years later, Price returned to Washington, Peters's adoptive parents finally obtained permission for him to come to the United States. Once in Pennsylvania he telephoned Price and was given a job at the Walter Reed Hospital. From there he moved to Case Western Reserve as senior technician with Dr. Kenneth Warren and so, firmly based in the New World, has worked ever since on the disease that came there via his own ancestral roots.

Pierre Peters has worked on schistosomiasis in such far-flung places as China, Egypt, and Kenya, and by now some people speak of him as "the most wanted man in schistosomiasis." The reason is simple: he has developed techniques that greatly speeded up the procedure whereby egg counts are estimated and thus a person's infection quantified. When he first visited St. Lucia with Kenneth Warren, now director of the Division of Health Sciences at the Rockefeller Foundation, these tests took ten days to complete and, to get accurate estimates, needed a back-up of laboratory facilities as well. Both men were worried about the time it took to test for infection and Warren suggested that Peters look into the matter. Soon he had developed a simple and cheap method for estimating the egg counts in a urine sample in a matter of minutes. When first tried in Kenya, the technique worked amazingly well; it was used to test two hundred children in just one day. Using knowledge that he had gained at St. Lucia, Peters next perfected an equally simple test for checking eggs in stools. It took him a mere two weeks to perfect this and both procedures are now routine ones recommended by WHO for field work. So not only has the time factor been sharply reduced, but the steps to be followed are so simple that local people can be easily and quickly taught, the results analyzed the same day, and errors in counting sharply reduced.

Dr. Adel Mahmoud, a consultant on the St. Lucia project, describes Mr. Peters in action:

When we travel, there is generally only Pierre and me, perhaps one or two more people – and soon we are starting to work with the local guys. Most of them don't speak English, but within ten to fifteen minutes Pierre has got a team of fifteen to twenty Egyptian assistants, or St. Lucians – just ordinary people – lined up into an assembly line and the testing system is going. In Egypt, we have examined two hundred samples of stools between nine o'clock in the morning and four in the afternoon. We have finished surveys in the field in weeks when people thought it would take months.

As the visitors to St. Lucia came and went, Pip Jordan presided over the entire sixteen years with a sure, calm touch. It is generally agreed that he did a remarkable job. A good leader who had the capacity to attract and keep good staff, he was an excellent administrator who kept to the protocols, ran a great show, and saw that his scientists published all the time. By background, character, and bearing, he fitted naturally and superbly into the place and the task.

Most of his colleagues came not only to admire but to love him, and when the program was completed the St. Lucians felt a terrible sense of loss and genuinely mourned the departure of the scientists, especially the man who had quietly kept the program on the rails, instilling confidence, and training many of them to take over those jobs that, in the normal course of events, they would never have had the opportunity to do.

Over and above this, Jordan's greatest contribution, Speed Unrau insists, was his ability to see the big picture:

We leaders of the various sections had our own projects, and each thought ours was more important than anyone else's. There were also conflicts of interest, but it was amazing how we were able to work so well together for so long, and how rapidly Pip learned. He felt initially that staff meetings might be a waste of time, since if anyone wanted to know what other groups were doing, all they had to do was to wander down to the laboratory and find out. Well, of course, no one did. So finally he called regular meetings and from then on we assisted each other in a whole variety of ways. Very often the hydraulic engineers could tell the biologists where they had spotted snails. Joe Cook spent days in the field with my group learning about the mechanics of water supply and the life patterns of people who might otherwise have ended up as patients in his clinic. And all the time Pip took care to see that a wealth of scientifically tested data poured out.

One hundred and sixty scientific publications emerged from this study. This by itself is no index of scientific quality, of course, but the peers speak of their meticulousness, the care and attention to detail, and how their conclusions are likely to hold for many years to come. For this research project is the only one in which the various methods of disease control have been scientifically compared and assessed. One scientist has gone on record as saying that not only is it unlikely that such a project will ever be attempted again in the foreseeable future, but if it were, it is unlikely that it could be successfully carried out. In 1981 Pip Jordan received the ultimate accolade, the George Macdonald Medal, an award given by the London School of Hygiene and Tropical Medicine, and the Council of the Royal Society of Tropical Medicine and Hygiene, for outstanding research leading to the improvement of health in tropical countries.

At the end of the entire sixteen years, the atmosphere took on the flavor of a children's party where everyone gets a present. Everything had worked, but each control method had advantages and disadvantages, and social and cultural influences could always scuttle strategies based on the most exquisite science.

The experience in Cul-de-Sac had shown that while control of snails can be highly effective, its success depends on a painstakingly detailed ecologic understanding of the population in every locality. Heaving chemicals into the water as a wholesale operation is a surefire method of poisoning the environment and wasting money, and since snails recover so rapidly from disasters, that job would have to be done continuously. What works superbly is careful applications of minimum quantities of chemicals, at those focal sites where humans meet water, but *only* if infected snails are present in that water. Since all these features will vary from one place to the next, only the principle – not the actual quantitative measurements – can be extrapolated from St. Lucia to countries like Egypt and Brazil. But so long as humans are passing eggs back into water a potential pool of infectious snails always persists.

Nonetheless there are some advantages to mollusciciding. Being dependent only on the labor of a few it requires a little cooperation from the many. It is thus independent of, and unaffected by, people's movements. But it takes several years to achieve an effect since even when diluted, the chemicals poison other life and so should never by sprayed in fishing waters. Finally, the cost of these compounds is steadily increasing.

Joe Cook's conclusions also contained good news and bad. Chemotherapy had come a long way from the twelve terrible daily injections to one, or at the most, two, pills taken by mouth just once a year. Oxamniquine has been used in five million persons so far with an outstanding record of safety, and its use is probably one of the largest examples of mass treatment with a single, modern therapeutic agent anywhere in the Third World. By now there are two other drugs and all, separately or together, provide cover for every variety of schistosomiasis infection that exists. Metrifonate, also manufactured by Pfizer, is taken orally in a single dose and its side effects are, WHO asserts, extremely rare. Praziquantel, manufactured by Bayer, is another cheap, safe drug, effective against all three species of parasite and can also be given in a single dose. Unlike the other two, we know how this one works: it interferes directly with the metabolism of the parasite. What other serious diseases can be effectively cured with one, or at the very most, two pills, once a year in a glass of water?

Even a miracle drug's potential to cure patients depends on an infrastructure that provides regular screening and treatment, however. Patients too must be cooperative if drug therapy is to be effective. There are two other disadvantages as well: a person can be cured and go straight back into a river and be infected all over again; second, it is difficult, as Joe Cook found, to achieve total coverage of a given population. He estimated that one-fifth of the people in his valley were untreated because that was what they wished and if such a percentage appeared in a program mounted with such dedication, in other circumstances probably 50 percent would remain untreated.

Finally there is no doubt whatever that fresh water is the best method for schistosomiasis control. Fresh water supplies work well only when supplemented with both laundry units and health education. The effect is not immediate and the system does little for those already ill. The major disadvantage relates to cost: since this solution to the problem is the most expensive, it is also the most unlikely. One massive, single capital sum is needed to pay for installation and further sums are needed for maintenance. Nonetheless as expensive as a water system may be, the St. Lucian experiment showed that the extra cost of communal laundries, shower units, and individual standpipes is minimal *and* brings maximum advantage.

Everyone agreed that this solution is to be preferred though, for in the period of simultaneous control measures, piped household water not only reduced new infections by 80 percent but brought other uncalculated benefits ranging from better growth and health of babies to a major reduction of gastrointestinal diseases in all the villages, to a dramatic reduction in the demands on physical energy that had been previously imposed upon the women. Thus in the late twentieth century, we are once more learning the lessons of the nineteenth: pure water supplies foster a dramatic improvement in public health. But, if the pun may be pardoned, it remains an open question whether the prospect is a pipedream or whether there is a real chance that this decade, identified by the United

Nations as the "Decade of Water," will see a dramatic improvement in this simple but vital health measure.

_____

Just what should we do, worldwide, for schistosomiasis? I returned to St. Lucia three years after my initial interviews with the project leaders to get the answers from the scientists themselves, for in April 1984, we all met up again. Joe Cook flew in from New York, where he now is program director of the schistosomiasis control program at the Edna McConnell Clarke Foundation; Mike Prentice flew in from Africa; I had already talked to Speed Unrau in Florida, Bob Sturrock in London, Fitzroy Henry in Bangladesh, and Peter Dalton in New York. Ken Warren, still at the Rockefeller Foundation, came down too and from the discussions I was able to see just what were the prospects for controlling this disease.

Though eradication is now no longer considered as a feasible target anywhere, the first thing I learned was that both the disease and the snail have practically disappeared from the island. I met a German doctor who had lived on St. Lucia for thirty years, and though this was only anecdotal reporting, he told me that when he had first arrived he regularly saw cases. But he hasn't seen a single one in a decade. This doesn't mean to say that no one is looking for schistosomiasis. They are, and for the snails too, for the procedures that the project teams devised to enable the St. Lucians to monitor the situation are still being faithfully followed.

Early one morning I joined two members of the staff, John Simon and Anthony Callender, to see schistosomiasis control in action. We were going to the Soufrière area, the locality where the disease had first been formally recorded and which used to have a high incidence. They loaded a Land Rover with their equipment – forceps, specimen bottles, and the "bible," written by the biology staff, a printed manual of procedures they would now follow if infected snails were found at the index sites. The manual listed work to be done on each day of a thirty-day schedule. They would read in the tables the amount of chemicals to be put in the water, in quantities that depend on the flow, which they first had to measure. Some tasks were "low priority," others "high," and the former could be canceled without danger if untoward events disrupted the routine.

It took us three hours to drive to Soufrière, through country dense with vegetation. At one point they stopped the van and, warning me to be careful because this was the area of the _fer de lance_, the most poisonous of snakes, showed me the rugged landscape they had once covered in the early surveys. It was impossible to see any people or houses and both had been very difficult to find.

Once through Soufrière we turned east into the hinterland to search the streams which fed the main river. One routine job is to clear debris from the flumes, metal devices placed at the sides of the streams, with a gauge that measures the flow and volume of the water. They cleared the first flume and drove two miles or so to another rough track where we parked again. John Simon led the way along the muddy path toward the river. As I moved toward the steppingstone he grabbed my arm and quickly pulled me back. It was not, as I had feared, a snake, but a large pile of shit.

Simon was livid. "Up here," he said angrily, "this is likely to be the Rastas. Local people now know not to use the streams as lavatories. But the Rastafarians cause us a lot of trouble. They want to go back to the forest and live with nature and they resist everything we do. They say we shouldn't treat the rivers and then they 'do their thing' straight into the water. It is not as if," he said in aggrieved tones, "we are constantly putting in chemicals. We only put them in if we find the right snails and if these snails contain larvae."

"Can you tell straight away whether they're infectious?" I asked.

"It's easy," said Simon. "We drop the snail in a little tube and hold it up to the sky. The light stimulates the cercariae to come out and the water becomes cloudy. Then we collect snails and take them back to the laboratory for microscopic examination and then return to put chemicals in the stream. But," he went on, "four Rastas were bitten by snakes last year and all died." The slight gleam in his eye suggested that he felt this just retribution.

We turned back toward Soufrière. About four miles out of town where the slope was easing, the two stopped to search for snails in another stream that fed the main river. They were actually looking for two kinds – the ones that carried schistosomiasis parasites and *Thira* snails, another species, which in the last few years had been introduced to displace them. These come from Dominica, are bred in the St. Lucian laboratory, and when introduced into the wild, reproduce so rapidly that they soon swamp other snail populations. Slowly they scanned twenty yards of the stream, a section where five months before two hundred fifty Thira snails had been introduced. They said that there were probably now four hundred Thira in just one ten-yard stretch.

Back to the Land Rover once more, and down another mile to the second station. Here the stream was wide and deep, so both men put on high rubber boots. While I waited, melting in the heat and humidity, they waded seven hundred yards downstream checking carefully. Gleaming forceps in silver patterns waved over the water; specimen tubes glistened from the tops of their pockets; the bright red of Simon's shirt stood against the green weeds as outraged ducks scattered in irritated splashes around their feet. But they found no snails.

Finally we went to the last checkpoint, a section of muddy sidewalks on the outskirts of Soufrière, along which little streams run which flood after the rains. On foot they checked around one block – a new block is covered each visit. Once more they found nothing, so we piled back into the Land Rover for the bumpy three-hour ride back to Castries.

"It has been like this for a long time," said Simon as he drove.

Back in the conference room on the Morne Simon's statement was amply confirmed by Mike Prentice. He had twice been asked back by the St. Lucia government to judge how the work was going, to see what had happened since the experiment finished, and to make new modifications to the control program in the light of worldwide improvements in techniques. When the scientists had departed, one of their greatest worries had been whether they would leave a total vacuum, so they felt that only the most simple, routine control measures would be likely to succeed. To their relief and delight, the recommended schedule of surveillance – which allowed the two-man team working five days a week to cover the entire island every six weeks and focus on known high-transmission areas – was generating remarkable results. Prentice explains the aims of the surveillance:

When I come back I am interested in two things – whether or not any infected snails have been found in our surveillance areas, and whether outside of these, there are a large quantity of the snails too. So far I haven't found any infected snails at all, but of course negative evidence is never satisfactory. I am quite certain that somewhere on the island there must be one or two infected snails about, and this is why it's very important that the surveillance must be continued for as long as possible. But the fact is that, whereas to begin with many infected snails were found in every scoopful of water or mud, now they are having difficulty in finding any at all, and this does point to considerable success.

So you can see it's very encouraging to realize that we've reduced the snail population by at least a thousandfold in the important areas, and in some areas by much more than that. There are some sites where they have been totally successful in eliminating the snail, where it has not been seen for four to five years. We were also very fortunate in being able to introduce the Thira snail, just at the right time, when people were placing emphasis on the chemotherapy and on the water supplies. So the disease was being forced back anyway, and the Thira snail added one extra push. But there is no question we have to keep a close eye on the situation, or the whole thing could revert.

In answer to the question, "In the light of what we now know, if snails were wanting to control schistosomiasis, would their target still be just everyone?" Prentice replied: "Not if they were as subtle as we now are. Their target would be to eliminate small boys." Joe Cook explained why. Small children had the greatest contact with water and this is true wherever schistosomiasis is found. They carry the greatest burden of infection and it is on them that the programs are now focused. Schistosomiasis infection peaks between the ages of five and fifteen, then for some unknown reason it drops by itself.

So all over the island, as well as at the Babboneau Health Centre in Marquis valley, five- to nine-year-olds are regularly screened. Pip Jordan may murmur nostalgically as he wanders around the empty laboratories, "These are where the biologists examined something like twenty-five thousand stools every year," with a dreamy, faraway look in his eyes. But now the children are screened by examining their blood, for the newest technique involves just fingerpricks of blood on filter papers. These are examined in London and are showing that there is no sign of renewed transmission on the island. "If this continues," Pip said, "then I think in a few years we will be able to say that there is virtually no schistosomiasis in the island."

It was Anthony Callender who took me to the Babboneau Health Centre, for that is his valley. We stopped the car by a dried patch of earth that provides the nursery, the training ground, for *the* game of the Caribbean: cricket. Two days earlier Pip and I had sneaked off to watch that lanky destructive giant of the West Indian cricketers, Joe Garner, slay some of Australia's finest batsmen in two successive overs, with balls that left his hand with a rocket's velocity. Since Callender is crazy about cricket and organizes games throughout the island, we had to watch as one small boy mimicked Joe Garner, while another mimicked the most famous batsman, Viv Richards. An argument developed as to whether Richards was out. "Come back on Sunday and play," invited John Simon. "The women play on Sunday." I said I would.

How easy and precise it now all was, I thought, as we left those lively, healthy children. Just as with mollusciciding, focal chemotherapy was turning out to be far cheaper, far easier to achieve, and more effective than a blanket treatment with pills. Hit the disease in young adolescents and blunt the highest peak of infection, and the amount of new schistosomiasis is sharply reduced. Such a selective approach is only possible because of the existence of the new, one-day-a-year drugs and the strategy is mass treatment of only that one target group. The aim is to get rid of 99 percent of their eggs, not to worry about the very last one, and this can be achieved with extremely low dosages.

The costs of both programs were low. To support the river surveillance cost only 75 EEC cents per person (that is, 25 U.S. cents), about $40,000 per year. To cure and protect the people in Marquis valley for the four years of intensive treatment had cost only $1.14 (U.S. $) per head.

I went to Richefond, of course, where clean piped water was still a huge success. People all over the island were still clamoring for laundries and shower units. Urban Glace took me to Grande Ravine and up to the pumping station for a close view of the notorious Thomazo tank. As the car crossed the bridge, marking the end point of a mile-long journey that the women of Grande Ravine used to make several times a day, there was no sign of anyone by the river. Up the hill, two small, naked boys were washing at their home standpipe, watched by an older girl about eight years old. The younger boy, about three, filled an enamel bowl with water. Bigger than his head, it took some lifting. Slowly he poured the water over his hair and the drops caught the sun as they fell. As we laughed I commented how clear the water was and Urban told me that the very first supply from the muddy meadow had contained iron and bacteria that left a red deposit. The people of Grande Ravine hadn't liked it. Proper water was clear and sparkling and they worried lest it leave a red deposit in their stomachs. But they had no complaints about their present supply, he said.

He was wrong. We passed the laundry where the only person working was a cheerful man, quite unperturbed at doing a woman's task, with a small baby in his care, perched on the slab of concrete between the sinks. But when Urban stopped at the point where the road bends sharply, a young, small, and extremely tough-looking woman thrust her head into the window of the car and spoke in patois. She then addressed me in English: "Do you know what I told him?"

"No," I replied.

"I said if the water doesn't come to my house, then repair the pipe!"

Thoroughly disconcerted at this public accusation of technical incompetence on the part of the Water Authority, the water supervisor just managed an embarrassed laugh.

"The water is good?" I asked the woman.

"Yes," she replied, "it's against bilharzia. They took my poop, lady. Do you know what poop is?"

I said I did. We drove slowly back down to the main road and as we passed the yard again the little girl was now as naked as her brothers. Noticing us see her, she froze into a statue of embarrassed delicacy, two tiny hands firmly placed over the parts that modesty insisted she hide.

Stupidly, I quietly said something to reassure her but she remained utterly immobile. Perhaps if she didn't move she couldn't be seen!

Finally we all met together and the scientists discussed the real point of the experiment, its relevance to the global situation in schistosomiasis. Pip Jordan emphasized that there would never be a single answer – no blueprint that could be applied throughout the world. Nonetheless, wherever schistosomiasis is endemic, the same four things are common: the parasite, a low level of sanitation, a snail, and its watery habitat. But while the pattern of contact with water is similar in places as far apart as Ghana or St. Lucia, Puerto Rico or China, there are great differences as to the snail and its habitat, and thus to the patterns of transmission. One study in Kenya showed that there major mollusciciding would have to be done every two months to keep the snail population down to a mere 5 percent of its original level. At other places spraying can hardly begin. Volta Lake in Ghana is an artificial lake of the type likely to be repeated many times as irrigation schemes spread. It is just not possible to control the snails where the shoreline extends for nearly four thousand miles! When the weeds to which the snails cling had been removed from certain spots, spraying certainly helped, but even when the disease was simultaneously being controlled by effective drugs, and good household water supplies, spraying had to be kept up once a month and the expense was formidable. In the irrigated parts of the Sudan, such as El Gezira, an area that has the potential for being the Florida of Africa, attempts to control the snail population seem equally fruitless. The fact that fifty thousand migrant workers are brought in each year to pick cotton does not help. They constantly reintroduce the disease and blanket mollusciciding seems not to have helped at all.

"But what about the Decade of Water?" I asked Pip Jordan.

As always political considerations impose their own imperative. It is important to remember, he said, that no government is going to bring in water to control schistosomiasis though they may do so for reasons that will range from the starkly political to a genuine concern for the health of their rural poor. Shortly after their project had ended, Jordan was very pessimistic about schistosomiasis control but now feels that the prospects are far rosier, for fast-moving events have overtaken the St. Lucia experiment.

Money, of course, will always remain a problem and what has been made available in the Decade of Water has fallen far short of what is needed to bring supplies to those people who desperately need them. The costs will be $30 billion a year for ten years, a formidable amount indeed but peanuts by comparison with other expenditures. Thirty billion dollars represents the world's expenditure on arms *every two weeks* and on tobacco every year; set against the current defense budgets of the United States or the Soviet Union the figures provoke impotent despair. However, money *is* being spent on water and sanitation, even if under other labels than schistosomiasis control. Many World Bank schemes, and other development programs like model villages, allocate 50 percent of their expenditures to rural water supplies, yet there is great variation from one region to another.

The Decade of Water is turning into a great success in Asia, arriving at just the right stage in the development of these countries, with most now ready to tackle water and sanitation. In India, where there is a major national plan, progress has been spectacular: one hundred thousand hand pumps are being installed every year and it is expected that there will be one in every village by the end of the decade. Pakistan, Thailand, Indonesia, the Philippines, and Sri Lanka too, are working toward the same end. Money is the only obstacle.

Shame can provoke a country to tackle this problem of water. At first Pakistan would do nothing, but when Mrs. Gandhi announced that India was undertaking to supply water on a countrywide basis, General Zia first called a national conference and then announced that Pakistan would too. Thus political realities are now playing into the hands of those who wish to improve public health, for governments are realizing that otherwise their own political systems may not survive. Fear is finally goading them into action. For example, Thailand is combating the "revolutionary conspiracies" (the government's phrase) with major programs to improve the quality of life in the northeast, and the same is true in southern Tunisia and in Sri Lanka.

The heart of Africa is another matter. No matter how it came about, Africa is a continent where many people are starving, on the verge of total economic collapse and political disruption, provoked by an equal mixture of ideology and incompetence, war and greed, circumstances and events. Schistosomiasis is rapidly increasing. There was none at all in Ghana before the dams were built; now 91 percent of Ghanaian children have the disease. For the moment there is little chance of implementing educational programs and developing in the African nations the professional skills needed to apply the scientific and technical solutions that research has given. Even where water projects have been successful, as in

India, we know so little about management and control, that, according to Nalni Jayal, adviser to India's Planning Commission, the country is nevertheless "on the verge of an enormous ecologic disaster. What is happening in Africa is going to happen in India within ten years." It is not that India is unlikely to meet its target providing clean water to every home by 1990. It will, but state officials everywhere are reporting that the supplies are drying up, and this is linked to the disappearance of forests as trees are cut for fuel. With the rains rushing straight down the hillside, the water disappears in uncontrollable floods. This is happening in Nepal, Thailand, and Malaysia, too.

Yet though water as an option for schistosomiasis control seems to be ruled out, paradoxically we can be optimistic, Pip Jordan insists. A press release on November 13, 1984, from WHO, tells why. A new revolution in control is already underway based on the method Joe Cook applied in the Marquis valley, and the talk is of bringing the disease down to levels undreamed of in the past. Why is WHO so confident? Safe and extremely effective drugs are one reason, and the low-cost diagnostic techniques easily used in rural areas, is a second. But, in addition, WHO claims that a "people-oriented" approach has already produced dramatic results in national programs, notably in Brazil, Egypt, and Sudan. By hitting hard at the heavier infections, the problem can be reduced to so low a level that it is no longer a public health problem.

In Sudan's El Gezira, where prospects once seemed perpetually gloomy, praziquantel supplied to adults and children has brought a drop in incidence from 50 percent to 11 percent. The minister of health for Sudan's central region, Mitamid Ahmed Amin, says, "There is no need for propaganda campaigns, the good news has spread fast. People are crowding into the centers, asking for the drugs." In the Nile Delta a campaign among schoolchildren similarly reduced the incidence from 90 percent to 13 percent, and among young people "a very high proportion of cases" are fully cured. In Brazil, where oxamniquine is being used, the situation is equally rosy.

Provided funds are available and coordinated efforts set up within the infrastructure to deliver the drugs, then progress could be rapid, even though major irrigation resource schemes come along in parallel. Funds will still have to be given by the mechanisms of outside aid, though, for the $1.14 per head that it cost to deliver the drug in the Marquis valley is still much too high for the developing world, where, in many countries, the total health budget is no more than $2.00 per head per year.

The last word, though, should go to someone who comes from a country where the problem is severe. Such a man is the Egyptian, Dr. Adel Mahmoud, chairman of Pierre Peters's department and a consultant to the St. Lucia project throughout.

In the final analysis development is going to change schistosomiasis. Don't forget that the distribution of the disease runs parallel to the social gradient of the society, and even in the smallest of villages in Egypt the rich can hire somebody else to get the water from the canal. They hire, in fact, someone to get schistosomiasis for them. It's not simply living in the countryside which determines whether you get the disease. It is who you are. So there are measures that we can achieve in the short run, and control by drug treatment is the most effective and the most important of these. But there are also measures we can achieve in the long run and the long run is obviously "development." In Egypt the well-to-do have just one or two children. But the people who can't feed themselves have twelve, and we can't say to them "Wait until development comes." Development is not just going to come. We have to work for it. So don't make the mistake of trying to take schistosomiasis out of the context of a society and what is happening in that society. You have to go back to its roots and decide upon a program of development and building for the people that is valuable – economically, politically and culturally – and somewhere in that package is schistosomiasis.

Thus the problem has subtly shifted. Science knows the cause of schistosomiasis, has tested the remedies in field trials, has developed an effective strategy that could reduce this infection dramatically in the years ahead. The problem is now political: there is no such thing as a simple technologic fix.

The St. Lucians consider themselves lucky that they provided the laboratory and the experiment. "I think that the last infected snails will be here after all the scientists have gone," said Anthony Callender as he scooped up mud in his routine search monitoring for the parasite's eggs. "No one is perfect, you know. But if the snail is hiding somewhere, I cannot find him. They are scared of me now because they are hiding from me. I have not seen one for five years." He put down his fishing net and prepared to take up his cricket bat.

4
The Last Outcasts

Only connect! That was the whole of her sermon. Only connect the prose and the passion and both will be exalted.

E. M. Forster, *Howard's End*

Before I went to Nepal my understanding of leprosy was similar to that of most people in the West. My knowledge was limited, my experience nil, and I wasn't especially keen to increase either. As a daughter of the manse I had first learned about leprosy when my parents showed me the small slits high above the nave in many English churches. In medieval times, when leprosy was common in Europe, such windows were the closest contact lepers could make with the congregation. Their scaly skins, thickened features, and eroded lips, fingers, and noses provoked revulsion and fear. By crying "Unclean," or sounding a bell, or wearing torn clothing, they were forced to identify themselves. Sometimes they were expelled from their villages or herded into special areas.

In modern times contributions for leprosy missions used to be a feature of Sunday collections, and so I learned that the disease was still present in other, not so fortunate, countries. Gradually, from other sources I acquire stores of misinformation, ignorance, and prejudice about the disease. It was widely believed that leprosy could never be cured; that it was so infectious and its victims so deformed that segregation was unavoidable; and that its consequences were so horrifying that only saintly missionaries were able to live with lepers. It was commonly thought that nothing could be done for these outcasts and the curse of Lazarus would remain forever on the face of the earth.

None of this is true. Most of us could live near leprosy without risk and we could easily control it any time we chose. For the first time in history its victims can face the future confident that their children will be free and they are the last generation of outcasts. The situation is finally changing. Nepal shows something of the world to come and in May 1984, just before the monsoon, I went there to see for myself. But to understand what is taking place, it is necessary to learn a little about Nepal and a lot about the disease.

Nepal is a buffer state between Tibet to the north and India to the south. In size, it is about the same as England laid on its side, for the distance from the Tibetan plateau to the plains of India is only 120 miles, while the distance across the country from east to west, is 400 miles. The northern border is marked by the ramparts of the high Himalayas, including Annapurna, Everest, and Kangchenjunga, peaks that rise to over twenty-five thousand feet. From this range fingers of hills point south toward India and their melting snows gouge out deep gorges and grand canyons, curtained by steep slopes, eroded and broken. Away from the high snows and the regions of rock and ice, the hills are wooded. The trees are rapidly vanishing though, as the desperate search for fuel drives people farther up the hillsides. The subsequent erosion is now a serious problem. Nepal is a landlocked country, but its special features make it really a series of islands. So steep are the slopes, so narrow the gorges, so fragile the paths, that an earthquake, landslide, avalanche, or flood can quickly isolate a region and keep it that way for weeks at a time. The paths are the tracks of the many tribal groups that make up the Nepalese, the two most famous being the Gurkhas and the Sherpas. In Nepal one is always walking uphill or downhill, so the people are wiry and lithe.

There are only two roads, one running north from the capital to Tibet and the second east-west from the Kathmandu valley, with a branch south through the foothills, and the jungle and forests of the border region where tigers still roam. From Kathmandu to Pokhara some three thousand feet lower to the east, takes no more than thirty-five minutes by airplane, but by road it can take five hours or more, and where roads are nonexistent communication is difficult and travel arduous. Though in recent years small aircraft regularly make flights up to high villages, their timetables are uncertain, since, as one pilot said, "Our clouds have rocks inside."

From the skies my first sight of Nepal was breathtaking, my first impressions enchanting. They never changed. The mixture of pride, independence, and friendliness, the prime characteristic of the happy, smiling Nepalese, was a constant joy. The old parts of Kathmandu, and the rural villages, reflect architecture of a style and structure that rivals anything medieval Europe produced. Strung along winding streets of dirt or stone, the houses are built of red clay bricks and are topped and faced with exquisite hardwood carvings, burnished under the rays of the sun. Myriad Buddhist temples and Hindu shrines exist, some high above flights of stone steps, others so small and intimate that one just stretches out to place a floating flower on its waters. The activity of farmers, merchants, *saraginhi**

---

* A Nepalese viola, constructed out of a single piece of hardwood, with an open resonance chamber, partly covered by drumskin.

players, and the porters pervades the streets. Women fetching water carry their infants along too; small children, brown and ragged, race around while adolescents trudge to school or herd the goats. Throughout, the sacred Bedu cows meander aimlessly down the thoroughfares and the stranger is greeted with the traditional *Namaste* uttered with the palms of the hands placed together and the head gently bowed.

As in St. Lucia, however, beneath the beauty, which is phenomenal, and the friendliness, which is total, poverty is universal. There are a few taps or standpipes in most villages, but each has also one, or more, ponds where the water is filthy black or dark green. In this, clothes and bodies are washed, animals drink, and children play. Where they exist at all sanitation arrangements are the simplest and it is difficult to achieve a high level of personal cleanliness. Moreover, medical facilities were minimal until recently, and in a country with steep hills and remote valleys, delivery of medical care is appallingly difficult.

This all bears on leprosy, yet when one thinks of the disease it is more tropical climes like India, Africa, the Philippines, or Brazil that come to mind. But the disease *is* a problem in Nepal and lepers are often seen. Though not known with accuracy, their numbers are likely to be as many as 100,000 in a population of 16 million, and are still rising. Most clinicians working in the country double the official estimates of 10 in every 1,000 people. Even though leprosy is considered to be a disease predominantly of warm areas it has been seen both in Nepal and Bhutan, among the people living at high altitudes, and as the surveys become more comprehensive, reaching farther into the remote areas, it is suspected that more cases may be found in the highest villages.

Leprosy is a chronic infectious disease that can take years to develop: it is caused by an organism similar to the one causing tuberculosis. Both diseases come from a group of mycobacteria that stain in a characteristic "acid-fast" manner, about forty species of which are known. How leprosy passes from one person to another is still not clear. How and where the bacillus actually enters the body is also not known, but we do know that the bacilli can survive for ten days outside their human hosts. Again as with tuberculosis, diagnosis starts with an examination of the skin, for the lesions begin as pale patches that have lost sensation. As the years pass other, more serious, effects appear, some resulting from enormous numbers of bacteria invading the nerves, while others, like burns, septic wounds, and ulcers, occur because the hands and feet become anesthetized or numb and injuries are no longer felt.

Though the mycobacterium was discovered in 1872 by a Norwegian, A. G. Hansen, and was also the first one to be implicated in a human infection, it still has not been cultivated in the laboratory, nor does any laboratory animal mirror human leprosy. Thus the search for a vaccine has been frustrated. Other characteristics made leprosy — also known as Hansen's disease — something of a clinician's nightmare: whereas most infection-causing bacteria divide at least once every twenty-four hours and thus provoke rapid symptoms, the leprosy bacillus takes nearly two weeks to divide, and symptoms can take years to show. The bacillus also has a predilection for certain sites, preferring body tissue that is cooler than the core temperature, usually the limbs, hands, feet, and nose. It can penetrate nerve cells that most other bacteria cannot and can thrive in the very cells of the immune system that are sent to destroy it, the macrophages. Worse still, since incubation can take from three months to thirty years it is impossible to identify infected people early, and physicians have no tests to reveal a subclinical infection of leprosy. Nor, until recently, was there any test to show whether a person had been cured.

On the bright side: not everyone is susceptible. It is rare for doctors or nurses in contact with patients to get the disease even after a lifetime of exposure, and few field workers have ever caught it. The sole exception was the famous Father Damien, the Belgian Roman Catholic missionary who ran the leper colony on Molokai in the Hawaiian islands and, after many years there, died of the disease in 1889. Many children born and bred in leprosariums have not contracted the disease, even though both parents had it. So most people are immune and several attempts during the last hundred years to infect volunteers have all failed. A mere 5 percent of people married to leprosy victims will contract the disease, and in southern India, where virtually everyone is exposed to the bacillus, only 4 percent of the population succumbs. Even a pair of identical twins can show differences of response.

Wherever leprosy is found, the reasons are the same. Nepal is a typical example — an extremely poor country, with simple systems of sanitation, inadequate health care, and a life that brings one into the closest contact with the environment. Feet walk on bare earth, for few houses have floors. Even in Europe where such conditions still exist, the disease is present in small pockets ranging through Portugal to Italy, Greece, Malta, and Turkey. In southern Spain, there are nearly four thousand registered patients and eight new notifications per year. Leprosy was rampant in Europe in medieval times. It did not begin to decline in England until the fifteenth century, in Denmark and southern Sweden until the sixteenth, and persisted in northern Scandinavia, Finland, Iceland, and along the eastern Baltic shores until the second half of the nineteenth century.

Nevertheless leprosy is once more on the increase and North America is no exception. A survey in 1982 showed that, in New York City, the number of new cases diagnosed each year during the 1970s was three times greater than in the previous decade. Ninety-nine percent of patients were foreign-born but had shown no symptoms when entering the United States, not unnaturally, for leprosy can take up to thirty years to appear.

Though it is in the tropics and the subtropical areas that leprosy still thrives, this has little to do with the heat or the humidity. Living conditions are the root of endemic leprosy. To dreadful poverty, appalling overcrowding, poor sanitation, few medical facilities, and little money to improve matters must be added malnutrition, parasitic diseases such as malaria, and constant infections, all of which overload the immune system and undermine general health. Moreover ignorance, prejudice, and other social factors make people reluctant to report their disease.

Worldwide there are now over five million registered patients (India alone has four million), but the total number is probably twelve million. Even though nearly 1.5 million patients have been successfully treated during the past ten years with new drug therapies, the gap between registered and suspected cases is primarily a consequence of the attitudes of healthy people. This is equally true in Nepal. Throughout the country, old people or those in the isolated high-altitude villages still believe people contract leprosy by drinking from the same well as a leper, or because they were wicked in a previous life, or that the disease is the result of a curse, witchcraft, or a visitation from the gods. Having no conception of how a disease can be caused by living organisms, they do not believe in the possibility of a cure.

This attitude is a relic of those found earlier, in Europe, ones that have not entirely vanished. Nepal has two such institutional reminders – the leprosarium at Khokana, some ten miles from Kathmandu, and another in the west. Khokana was founded more than sixty years ago and all patients were forcibly banished to this remote area above one of the rivers feeding the Kathmandu valley. A small clinic, merely a couple of rooms, is flanked by a small garden at the bottom of which is an even smaller schoolhouse where the young children are taught. The main accommodations are simple rooms in the three-storied buildings set round a central courtyard with its banyan tree, shrine, and temple, where daily offerings are made. Many of the inmates have lived here for years. The most up-to-date treatment is given at the weekly clinics, but still these people, some of whom came here when they were very young, eke out their lives in this fossilized place. Most would not want to leave; like long-term prisoners or mental patients, most are too scared to relinquish the only security they have ever known and reenter a world that was bitterly hostile when they left. One such man is an Indian schoolteacher, Kissan Singh Master, fifty-seven years old, who was admitted to the leprosarium twenty years ago. He had contracted leprosy when seventeen and was in the Leprosy Hospital in Almoora in India when a friend told him of how the Nepalese were trying to bring every support – physical and psychological – to leprosy patients. So he came north to Khokana, where he married, and here his son was born. Though his whole family are surrounded by leprosy, only he has the disease. On vitamin and drug therapy, he teaches in the school and seems completely satisfied with his life. "We get everything from the government," he says, "rice daily, water and tea, soap, wheat and barley, and weekly visits from the doctor. Here we live; here we are happy and safe."

But no one else will ever again be admitted to Kokhana and the government looks forward to the time when the two leprosariums will close, for this will mean that leprosy is being successfully treated *within* the community. These hospices are a tremendous drain on the government's few resources, taking money away from programs that are one hundred times more valuable for leprosy control. But the government cannot and will not force these people to leave. This sad place, safe haven yet life in limbo, embodies all that is wrong with old attitudes to leprosy – the isolation, handouts, lifetime support, passive acceptance, lack of expectations, and resignation that drains away initiative. All such attitudes will have to change, and they will too, when the real nature of leprosy and what can be done are fully understood by the people.

Poor though it is, Nepal is tackling its problems with vigor. The chief of the country's Leprosy Control Project, Dr. R. B. Adiga, described their plans as follows: The country has been divided into fourteen zones and at least one referral center will be set up in each region. Two already exist; the central region is overseen by the Anandaban Hospital, run by the Leprosy Mission; in the west near Pokhara, another mission, Green Pastures Hospital, is also a referral center. These referral hospitals shelter leprosy patients who require institutional care. But the majority do not require such care, and as education and treatment progress, fewer and fewer will have to be hospitalized. So a series of nine community health centers will be established, but not for leprosy alone. They will treat *all* communicable skin diseases and will ultimately amalgamate with the general hospitals.

Nepal being a country of vast distances, leprosy victims may have to walk for twelve days to obtain treatment; as a rule they simply will not do this. The priorities of a man living high under Annapurna or Everest are food for his family first, looking after his animals second, with his disease low down on the list. But if leprosy is to be controlled he must be regularly examined and treated, so the clinics must go to him. Thus the core of the programs will be mobile teams, so structured that a few trained people serve many. Ideally each team will have a medical officer, a nurse, physiotherapists, other technicians to take diagnostic smears, orderlies, and drivers. But this is all for the future. At the moment control relies on the paramedics already at work and in two separate excursions I was taken to see what they do.

Pokhara is a small town that is the main trekking center for Annapurna. Five miles outside Green Pastures is the German mission station, responsible with the Nepalese government for western Nepal. Here the paramedics receive their training and, on a regular schedule, fan out into the surrounding districts. Inevitably the place is well away from the villages and reached via stony tracks over fields. Beside the hospital and living quarters for the doctors and visitors is a building where the paramedics receive instruction. The leader of their team is a young man aged twenty-five who has worked in the leprosy program for over six years. He is highly intelligent and deeply committed; he needs to be, for it takes real stamina and a strong stomach to be a paramedic in this program. The work is exacting and hard, starting at sunrise and returning home as late as ten at night, having driven over a hundred miles on appalling tracks. A team I walked with had, only two weeks before, trekked for nineteen hours one day to find a patient, not reaching him until two o'clock the next morning. There are severe psychological demands on the paramedics too, for old attitudes die hard; when a paramedic walks out from his village people will murmur, with interest always, dismissiveness regularly, and fear sometimes: "He's going to the leprosy hospital." The medical authorities recognize these problems and try to give the paramedics a mixture of incentives, including reasonable food and comfortable lodgings, as well as ensuring that their morale is kept up by praise, job security, and by training skills to qualify them to tackle other medical conditions. Still, in terms of social acceptance it is far easier for a foreign missionary to work in leprosy than for the Nepalese themselves.

A typical excursion was the trip I took with seven young paramedics to a small settlement to make an educational presentation on leprosy. The village rests on a spur of land running alongside a deep gorge. Its center is the ubiquitous banyan tree and shrine, and houses and tea shops are strung along the main path. Children surged round as the vehicle drew up, watching as the team began tacking posters on the tree trunks and shop walls and placing fliers in outstretched hands. Many of the fliers would end up as paper darts, or as wrapping paper, but not all. Then the seven pied pipers climbed over a small wall, and led the way to an open field, drawing some men, many women, and most children after them. There were at least a hundred youngsters; the process of educating them and reeducating their parents was the aim of the exercise.

When silence had been more or less restored, dogs shooed away, and crying babies suckled, the meeting began. The leaders said that leprosy was not a result of a visit from the gods or any other such reason but had one simple cause: it was an infectious disease just like syphilis, colds, or fever. It was not contagious and therefore there was no reason to throw victims out of the community. Since the disease could be now cured they should encourage their friends to go to the referral centers or report to the paramedics. It was vital to recognize the symptoms early, and later, one of his colleagues would describe these, for the earlier the disease was diagnosed, the better the cure and the less the likelihood of deformities. A patient must stay through the entire length of treatment, for then cures could be guaranteed.

Another paramedic described the clinical signs and the simple diagnostic tests and a third explained the protocols of treatments and where the drugs could be obtained. After twenty minutes the audience was flagging, but then a fourth paramedic stepped up to tell the children a story. Holding some ten simple, but charming, large line drawings, he began: "Once upon a time." Everyone in the audience sat up; glazed eyes brightened, and raptly they followed, alternately sad and laughing.

Once upon a time there was a small boy who lived with his family and developed leprosy. His father took him to the village Brahmin who ordered him to leave. Weeping bitterly the boy walked to the nearest town, where he was forced to beg. As they could see, he was unhappy, destitute, and very lonely.

One day paramedics visited the boy's village, and a friend of his became convinced that leprosy can be cured. So the friend went in search of the leper boy and fortunately was successful in finding him. He persuaded the boy to go to the clinic, and after six months' treatment the little leper was finally cured. So together they returned home, where the banished boy showed his father how he was able to work, and so could help support the family.

The story has a happy ending of course, and it had an ironic epilogue. For the Brahmin himself develops symptoms of leprosy and it is the boy whom he banished who takes him to the clinic. So all lived happily ever after.

There was no sound while the story was told, only the distant bleat of the odd goat and the calls of the birds. Then questions were invited and there were a few lively exchanges: Was the disease inherited? Why did some people catch it and not others? Who would pay for the drugs? Finally pills were distributed to those patients already under treatment. A few suspected victims were examined and then the gathering dispersed and everyone wandered back across the field and into the square.

Surrounded by children, we ate our sandwiches. Then with cheers from the youngsters and *Namastes* from the adults we were off, with small boys chasing the Land Rover for as long as they could keep up. As we turned the corner, leaving the village behind, a water buffalo could be seen stolidly munching a leprosy poster that a paramedic had stuck onto a tree.

Two weeks later, in central Nepal, a second group of paramedics demonstrated other aspects of the work. They were going to pay a house call on a patient, but he lived many miles from the overnight rest stop, three valleys and several thousand feet away. Once more, we all piled into the Land Rover very early in the morning. Besides the paramedics there were now three local porters to carry food and medical apparatus — stains, glass slides, pills, bandages, needles, scalpels — in the large woven baskets. These are carried on the back, but their triangular weight is supported by headbands crossing the forehead, an arrangement that can, over the years, make a perceptible dent in the bones of the skull.

After two hours, lurching, climbing all the time, the vehicle came to a halt, for the road went no farther. I was shown the valley which we had to descend and the distant final ridge we would have to climb. The patient was some way beyond. A gentle track running off to the left was ignored, as suddenly the four paramedics disappeared over the edge, aiming straight for the opposite ridge. In the next few hours' trek, the paramedics and the porters danced down the tracks and flew up the slopes. It was easy enough to the valley floor, exciting to cross a single log over a stream, delicious to rest and drink at the teahouse. But then began the unrelentingly steep climb up the other side, and as my heartbeat quickened my pace slowed. The team climbed on and on – it seemed that the ridge would never appear – but suddenly we reached the top of the pass at nine thousand feet, and they burst into song.

"What are you singing?" I asked them, between gasps.

Bisha the senior paramedic answered: "It's a traditional Nepalese song they sang: 'Pretty lady, I have come to your house and you are going to invite me to drink tea. But quite frankly I would prefer to take you to the forest.'"

"And how does it end?" I asked.

They all looked horribly embarrassed. "We couldn't possibly tell you that," they replied.

A slim, white-coated figure now appeared over the skyline, the paramedic who had gone ahead to tell the patient that the team was coming. It was premonsoon season and the weather was humid and sticky, the leeches in full force. Because of the rain the high mountains had been obscured for days, but suddenly it was as if a curtain had been drawn. Even at a distance of thirty miles, the parting of clouds was exhilarating as the ramparts of the Himalayas burst out of the clouds at 45° up, sentinels of the top of the world.

The patient, Man Singh, was in his late fifties. He was a fine figure of a man with an aquiline nose and must have been strikingly handsome in his youth. He had developed leprosy in 1962 and was put on the only effective drug then available, dapsone. He defaulted from treatment for one year but then reappeared and since 1981 has been on the new drug regimen. Man Singh was doing very well, according to senior paramedic Bisha, who said, "We did a skin smear on him in February 1982 and it was completely negative. So the therapy is working and I expect this smear to be negative too."

To do an initial diagnosis of leprosy, the paramedics search the skin for the white patches that suggest an infection and are numb. If such patches are found, they are touched with a needle while the patient, with closed eyes, tries to indicate the needle's position. One paramedic now grasped Man Singh's ear, swabbed the lobe, and neatly slit the skin with a scalpel. He smeared the tissue over the slide, waved it to dry, then applied the stain. In the laboratory, the slide would be scanned for the mycobacteria that show up as red rods.

Everyone was crowding round, but the patient appeared relaxed and there was no sign of any rejection, either of him or his family. Asked whether it was the case that the farther from Kathmandu the greater the superstition and the paramedics' difficulties, Bisha replied:

"Well we don't actually tell them that we've come to test for leprosy. We tell them that we have come to examine skin diseases, whether bacterial or parasitic. Then we do a general survey of a whole village, and if we find a person with anesthetic fingers or feet, we don't tell them straight away that they've got leprosy. That would worry them. We ask them to come to the clinic and there we do the final investigations. When we are quite sure we tell only the person. We don't even tell their relatives.

There is still a stigma [in remote areas], but so long as they have good hands and feet they are not worried. If they are badly deformed and horrible looking, then certainly they can be neglected. Since they are not infectious, they do not harm the community, but still the community doesn't like to keep them. As long as they are without the deformity, they can still be highly infectious yet nobody seems to mind.

As he watched his other colleagues examine the children, Bisha then spoke of the great distances the paramedics had to cover on foot to reach their patients, "We're responsible for an area that takes four days to cross. We can't carry much food, and there are no tea shops along the way, so we can walk hours and hours without eating anything. But the people are very kind and if they see us they try to provide something. Sometimes we will go a whole day just eating a piece of bread made in the villages."

By now his colleagues had finished with Man Singh. His bone-crushing handshake showed how strong his hand still was, unlike un-treated lepers' hands, which are often clawed and deformed by the disease. After one hour the group retraced its steps.

The poverty of Nepal affects leprosy in a large number of ways besides affecting the incidence of the disease. The resources of any country with a low gross national product are bound to be quite inadequate for disease control, so Nepal has to turn to the outside for help. The proud and independent nation would dearly love to manage alone, but unfortunately, such dependence is inescapable. Many separate missions set up hospitals and stations in Nepal, and while these retain a certain autonomy, nevertheless they are now all closely incorporated into the country's programs. They undertake specific projects but are totally responsible for referral and control in different areas of the country. The Anandaban Hospital is one such center and is part of a series of hospitals run by the Leprosy Mission in thirty-four countries. This international and inter-denominational mission has its headquarters in London, and maintains

148 centers, conducts 2,399 clinics, and provides care for approximately 300,000 leprosy patients all over the world.

To get to Anandaban one must go south from Kathmandu. No more than five miles as the crow flies, it is forty minutes as the Land Rover lurches. It was harvest time and the main streets of three ancient villages along the way were crammed with wheat being stacked, threshed, winnowed, and sacked. Clear water gushed from a few standpipes, but black water stagnated in the ponds. Once through these villages the road climbs steeply on a track that is a quagmire of mud in the monsoon. Following across the flanks of three hills, it rounds hairpin bends and as the valley floor falls away below so wooded hills approach from above. Between is red sandstone country, with terraced slopes of wheat and rice, where a telltale fire periodically reveals the illegal burning of a forest patch being cleared for crops.

Then the road abruptly shifts east, drops down, and runs along a small and very beautiful valley. Now neither Kathmandu nor its valley can be seen and this was intentional. For when in 1957 the Leprosy Mission was invited by the Nepalese government to begin leprosy control activities, isolation and remoteness were still the norm. The road was cut in 1958, and staff headquarters and a patients' block were built the following year. Not only was the hospital placed far away and unsuspected, but the buildings deliberately present their backs to the capital, even though they couldn't be seen anyway, for a high hill blocks Anandaban from the Kathmandu valley.

The road swings up to the Mission in a series of bends. The white buildings, stacked up the hill, merge into a landscape of eucalyptus and pines like a university campus in northern California. The final driveway of hand-laid stones moves up from the research laboratory to the living quarters, to the main administrative building and surgical unit. Above are the men's wards, the women's wards, and the outpatients' department. The birds singing from the trees splash trails of color as they dash across the sky; there are six hundred species in Nepal. Flowers grow all over in gardens lovingly tended by ex-patients who have never wanted to leave. Slim nurses, dressed in long, dazzling white gowns, with their single badge of professional qualification the only decoration, walk serenely from ward to ward. The shoemakers, as leathered as the hides they work, squat in the sun outside their shop, making comfortable sandals from old motor tires and water buffalo leather. The name of the place, Anandaban, means "forest of joy," and it is apt.

If Nepal is a microcosm of leprosy problems worldwide, Anandaban is a microcosm of problems in Nepal. On this quiet campus one can see and experience the range of challenges that leprosy presents, medical, scientific, and spiritual challenges. Anandaban is not just a place of healing, it is a place of research and of teaching, a place whose activities embrace the whole of the leprosy patient, their present treatment, and their future hopes.

Dr. Narsappa Matthew Samuel and his wife, Dr. Susie Samuel, run Anandaban, with the help of nurses, paramedics, shoemakers, technicians, porters, nightwatchmen, drivers, dhobie (laundry) men, physiotherapists, cooks, and all. Known to everyone as Sam and Susie, he is forty-six, she forty-two. A clinical specialist in leprosy and a research scientist, he is superintendent and director of the hospital; she is physician and surgeon. Sam comes from Hyderabad in the middle of India, where his father was a Methodist minister. Susie's father was an Anglican canon in Singapore, but the two met at college in India. Married in 1971 they have two children at school in India. Sam had always intended to work in leprosy and specialize in rehabilitative orthopedic surgery. But while doing his final year at St. Mary's Hospital, London, he met a pioneer in leprosy, the British doctor, Stanley Browne, who told him that if he wanted to control leprosy, it was not surgery he should be doing, but clinical medicine, and prevention as well as treatment.

Both convinced Christians, the Samuels joined the Leprosy Mission shortly after their marriage. They were first posted to Bhutan, that remote Himalayan kingdom on the northwest frontiers of India and Pakistan. After three years they asked for study leave and went to London. While Narsappa Samuel took his Master of Science degree, doing a thesis with Dr. John Stanford, a bacteriologist and immunologist at the Middlesex Hospital, Susie Samuel completed her training in obstetrics and gynecology. When the year was over the Leprosy Mission told them that there was an opening in Nepal and asked if they were interested. They were indeed, but as the airplane landed Susie burst into tears: "You have brought me to another isolated mountain," she said.

The first years were not easy, for they had to expand the hospital and build the laboratories from scratch. Initially the staff numbered thirty, but in five years it rose to seventy-six and the budget trebled. Equally important, the Samuels began to undertake research projects; they speak with warm gratitude of the understanding of the Leprosy Mission, originally hesitant to back research. The hesitation arose because the Mission is a service-oriented organization, and benefactors who give money for leprosy like to feel that it is going for patients. But Sam belongs to a famous tradition of scientists who firmly believe that it is the juxtaposition of patient and laboratory that provides the best opportunities for discovery of clues to disease and for an immediate impact on treatment.

The visitor to Anandaban soon comes to see how it is that one of the oldest of human diseases could now be controlled if society so chooses. But though scientists and doctors, pharmacists and immunologists have provided us with the tools to do this job, it still remains unfinished.

Apart from the beauty of the place and the joyous warmth of the welcome and the intelligent discussions of the problem with two committed scientists who are devout, unstuffy, and amusing people, what strikes the visitor immediately is the sheer joy of the place. Anandaban is a hospital run like any good hospital anywhere but with one special difference: everything is geared to making the patients feel wanted. Everything is focused not only on helping them forget the many terrible things that may have happened before, but on curing, securing, and sustaining them so that they can return to the world that previously rejected them. Thus Anandaban straddles two worlds – the past and the future – a fascinating stance as subtle shifts in social attitude are rapidly coming together with new tools in science. The situation is changing so quickly that the world's next generation may not remember how appalling the situation once was for lepers.

From the world of the past are patients who were caught too late, whose long-term treatment is difficult, and whose social rehabilitation will be impossible. Ram Baradur Lama is in his middle years but looks much older, bewildered and lost. Banished from his village when he caught the disease, he was abandoned in the jungle, his wife having committed suicide. After he had lived alone in the jungle for eleven whole years, someone discovered him and took him to Anandaban. But, by then, his untreated leprosy had progressed so far that he was badly deformed. He is now regularly treated, well looked after, feels marginally more secure, but neither his body nor his life can ever be adequately reconstructed.

Shanta Maya stands squarely in the intermediate group, between past attitudes and future hopes. She comes from the region of Kangchenjunga in eastern Nepal. No roads connect with Kathmandu, only miles of narrow paths. Steep valleys and deep gorges separated her from the only place where she could get treatment. She was married, with three sons, when she developed symptoms of leprosy; the elders of the village threw her out and her husband remarried. They gave her a rough shack, the size of a pigsty, some distance outside the village, and told her to leave. She pleaded for at least one child to be with her, and her youngest son, Shaila, was allowed to go. Shanta Maya had no intention whatever of giving up, so together they walked to Kathmandu, taking fifteen days, begging for food and shelter as they went. By the time they arrived, the ulcer on her leg was so fiercely inflamed and infected that, in agonized pain, she could hardly stumble along. Once in Kathmandu they asked for the general hospital but even after directions it took them three days to get there. On arrival at the hospital she was immediately referred to Anandaban. Somehow they made their way, but as soon as Dr. Susie Samuel saw the leg she knew it would have to come off. She told Shanta Maya that they would take her back to Kathmandu for the amputation.

"No sooner did we get her into one door of the Land Rover," recalls Susie, "then she opened another and hopped out. So we put her back in and she came out again on the opposite side. This happened three times and finally she said she didn't care if she died here, but go back to Kathmandu she would not. It was pure blackmail," she adds with a chuckle. "Now I had never done an amputation before in my life, but what could we do? I said 'All right, we'll amputate your leg tonight,' and did it at 11:30, and this was my first amputation."

Eighteen months later that courageous, laughing woman is hopping about on her artificial limb like a mountain goat. Her son, proud of his mother, also has quiet pride in himself, and everybody is devoted to them. They were soon to return to their village. A few years before some New Zealanders had visited Anandaban and left enough money for one patient each year to be given a water buffalo. These two were to receive the "Water Buffalo Award for 1984." The animal would either be taken back with them or bought in their area; the Samuels would see this was properly organized. Once back in the village, with her disease cured and her deformity compensated, the mother and her devoted son would have wealth and status. They could hire out the water buffalo to plough, sell its milk, and could use its dung for fuel. So unlike patients at Khokana, not only can they be encouraged to go back, but they want to go back.

Those who truly know they can be cured represent the future. They come for treatment, early and voluntarily, always intending to return. Bhim Prasad, in his midthirties, lives at the western end of the kingdom of Nepal. He contracted leprosy and soon the characteristic clawed hands marked him as a victim. As the disease begins to affect the nerves, the muscles fail to receive messages and become wasted, so the fingers are gradually pulled in toward the palms. One day, without a word to his wife, Bhim Prasad left. When he turned up at Anandaban Hospital he was put straight onto drug therapy and shortly after, in her tiny surgical suite, Susie operated on his right hand. Under local anesthetic a less important tendon in the wrist is split into four. The four strips of slit tendon are slid beneath the skin and grafted into place at the tip of each finger, connected to the appropriate muscles, for each will be made to perform the function of the damaged tendons that normally control movement and grip. After six weeks in plaster the tendons and the muscle are retrained by the resident physiotherapist to work together with the brain. Bhim Prasad, thrilled with his new right hand, is shortly returning home to show his wife that he is cured and his hand functioning. Eventually he will return to have the operation on his second hand.

Goma Bandari too came of her own accord. In her early twenties, she developed symptoms shortly after she was married and this landed her in trouble with her mother-in-law. "Mothers-in-law make or break marriages in Nepal," Susie commented. Goma has received surgery and though she will never recover feeling in her fingers they look normal again and that, she considers, is the miracle that saved her marriage. Rameysh, too, the trapeze artist and circus clown, is a volunteer-outpatient in the clinic. Not only did he have a marriage to save but a job as well and the warmth and security of his circus family. "Though I wouldn't have liked to be at the other end of the trapeze from him before he came to us," comments Susie. His hands have now been restored, his illness treated, and he is progressing really well. He caught the disease from his wife who also gave it to their young daughter. But all three are receiving drug therapy and, Rameysh reports, his friends in the circus were so happy to have him back, working again in the ring where he continues to convulse everyone.

Anandaban receives some patients from hundreds of miles away, from all social groups, and there is a rather complicated social reason for this, which Sam explained.

You must understand that this institution was one of the first set up in the country and anyone who developed leprosy tried to come, for we would always admit them. Now with greater emphasis on outpatients and home treatment, people have swung too much perhaps to the other side, saying we don't need hospitals and we don't need beds for leprosy. When a person feels really sick they like to sleep somewhere and when they have a serious medical problem, they like care, and I am sure that this is one reason why compliance with the drug regimen has not always been 100 percent successful. So people are still coming. We used to do a clinic in Jungla – in the mountains in the northwest. Our doctors would fly in a chartered aircraft, do a clinic and then return here. Some bureaucrat said "It's too far and too expensive," so they stopped the flying clinic. But the patients in western Nepal still relate to Anandaban and in winter, from October onward, we have plane loads of patients flying in. They are rich people, farmers who may have a lot of sheep, and come on their own. They get admitted and we feel a little concerned for we just can't discharge them. So we keep some of them for six months or even one year, until we have at least completed 50 percent of their drug therapy.

As secure, comforting, and necessary as the hospitals may be, for clinicians and scientists they represent defeat, for none of the traditional deformities associated with leprosy are inevitable now. Certainly though, doctors yearn for a test that could identify patients early and public health instruction that would alert them to come in quickly. Best of all, they dream of a short and effective treatment for leprosy like the single, annual pill for schistosomiasis. But their ambitions are not cosmic; the present tools are remarkably effective if the patients are treated in time, and by contrast with the past, present therapeutic prospects are excellent.

To understand why the new drug protocols are so successful, it is necessary to understand the nature of a leprosy infection and its clinical course. It is far more complicated than one might imagine. At their out-patient clinic in the new general hospital of Patan, ten miles from Kathmandu, each Tuesday the Samuels see a sample of that 4 percent of the population who cannot resist a leprosy infection. The use of the dermatology clinic in a general hospital is something quite new and strikingly daring in leprosy control, all part of the campaign to remove the barriers between the patients and everyone else. As in Anandaban, many find their own way to Patan. Hearing of a possible cure they may struggle for days, walking over the mountains on diseased limbs; others are carried in on the backs of relatives. Others come to collect supplies of their daily drug and receive the supervised once-a-month dose of a second drug, and some come for physiotherapy. Most important of all they now bring along members of their family, or friends, for check-ups.

There are two types of leprosy, each dictating a specific treatment. In the minor form, only a very few bacilli are around and though they do gain entrance to the body's cells, eventually the body mounts an immune response. Unfortunately though, this is often less than perfect; in fact it's half-hearted. One consequence is that in the process of killing the bacteria, the immune cells also damage innocent bystanders, the nerve cells, by stripping off their sheaths. These cells can be damaged for another reason too, for the leprosy bacillus is one of the few organisms that can live inside nerves. As they increase in number, and the defending immune cells pile into the site, the whole area swells. The normal tissue first becomes grossly distorted, then permanently damaged, by the sheer pressure of invading cells. When this process occurs inside a myelinated nerve, a broken nerve and irreversible damage result. So whether the immune response affects the nerve, or whether the invading bacilli do, sensation is killed in that area with the result that subsequent injuries or trauma go unnoticed. The tissues turn septic and as infection spreads, a gangrenous mass follows, leading to the dropping off or amputation of the fingers or toes. Paradoxically, those people with the grossest deformities, whose lurid nature always caused revulsion in the onlookers, are those who not only actually are not infectious but probably *never* were. Their condition, paucibacillary, meaning few bacilli, is *tuberculoid leprosy.* Relatively few leprosy germs are in the system, and with sustained treatment a patient can be cured in six months.

At the other end of the spectrum are patients who, though highly infectious, look perfectly healthy, apart from a glossy, puffy look to their face. They are walking cultures of leprosy bacilli, swarming with active leprosy germs. A skin smear stained on a slide will reveal a mass of tiny red rods growing together in characteristic clumps of up to fifty bacilli at a time. The clinical problem they present is formidable. If they remain untreated, the infection leads to facial damage, the nose collapses, and the eyebrows disappear. This form of disease is called *lepromatous leprosy,* and this is where the real problem lies, for these patients are the only ones who can die of the disease and are the ones who spread infection. The bugs ooze from the skin: there can be ten million of them in the nasal secretions. In those places where people don't eat with knives and forks but dip with their hands into a communal pot the infection spreads quickly through a family. People can be cured but only if they are treated for two years continuously.

Between these two extremes all intermediate ranges appear, which makes it difficult to determine a patient's status and predict how the disease will develop. An untreated tuberculoid patient can become lepromatous; in a lifetime one person may swing drastically from one extreme of the disease to the other, or oscillate between. If no treatment is given, or if treatment is mismanaged, the disease will erupt time and again: the patient will suffer recurring spasms of reaction and agonizing nerve pain.

The success of treatment is monitored by the same test that confirms the diagnosis, the slit-skin smear test. It is often repeated at three-monthly intervals for two years, and if the regimen has been followed correctly, then gradually the bacilli become fragmented and eventually may disappear altogether. This always seems to happen with tuberculous patients. But in the lepromatous form, even though the lesions settle down and generally the patient does so well that it can often be difficult to see just where the lesions once were, not all the bacteria may have gone. At present there is an argument among the specialists as to whether only dead bacteria now remain or whether some living ones still do. Since in severe lepromatous cases the disappearance of every single bacillus from the skin can take years, the Samuels do not feel justified in terminating treatment for these patients even after the recommended two years. It is well worth persisting, however. For if a paucibacillary patient is successfully treated, this is a cure for just one individual; but if the infectious, multibacillary, patient is treated, then this is a lasting success for the whole community.

Of the three drugs currently in use, dapsone has been such a favorite that it formed the backbone of leprosy treatment for forty years. Effective and cheap, the bottles in which it was packed were often more expensive than the drug itself. But though they worked, the consecutive doses of gray pills did not show dramatic effects, so some patients got bored and did not take treatment regularly. Others failed to take the pills at all. Still others, arguing that if one pill does you good the whole monthly dose would be even better, swallow the lot in one go and suffer dire effects. In any case there is an almost inevitable pattern to therapy in poor countries, one that leads to drug resistance. Low dosages of a single drug is one element, but so too are irregular and inadequate treatments, lack of compliance, lack of medical supervision, and only intermittent availability of the drugs. The more poorly managed a control program, the more likely that drug resistance will develop. Resistance to dapsone surfaced only too soon. First noticed in 1964 in laboratory mice, it was soon reported from all parts of the world and in Nepal is a big problem. Unfortunately the effects are not limited to the individual patient. As those with dapsone-resistant disease relapse, their condition becomes multibacillary, they begin to infect others, whose disease is resistant to dapsone from the start. The World Health Organization soon realized that a crisis point was approaching worldwide, and something new was urgently needed.

Two other drugs are now used in combination with dapsone, in a recommended protocol called multidrug therapy (MDT for short). In this the old chemotherapeutic agent, dapsone, is combined with a red dye, clofazimine, and a derivative of a fungus, rifampicin, in a carefully directed and well-timed protocol. The discovery of these last two antileprosy agents, developed and marketed by Ciba-Geigy, is a unique illustration of just what an odd process discovery in science can be. It illustrates that the same logic can sometimes work for you and sometimes against you.

Since leprosy and tuberculosis are caused by bacilli from the same group, it seemed logical to expect that a drug effective against the one would prove equally effective against the other. Lamprene, the trade name for the red dye clofazimine, was jointly developed as an antituberculous drug by Vincent Barry and his colleagues at the Irish Medical Research Council at Trinity College, Dublin, and Geigy. It successfully cured mice of tuberculosis, but the results in humans were disappointing. The staff at the pharmaceutical company, faced with making commercial quantities, were not too unhappy when they learned that Lamprene seemed to be ineffective. They didn't relish the task of getting the stuff into a form suitable for clinical administration, for it could neither be compressed into tablets nor rolled into pills. Those working on the problem stood out in a crowd, for the bright red powder dusted them from head to toe. One sneeze would send it all over the room and when a flask was once accidentally dropped, an entire laboratory had to be redecorated.

Given the failure against human tuberculosis, logic dictated no trial against leprosy. Yet oddly enough, the first laboratory tests in 1958, by Dr. Chan at the National Institutes of Health in Maryland, were most promising. Once again, however, it was still possible that what worked in mice might not work in men. In 1960 human trials were arranged with large volumes of the drug being supplied free of charge; the results were excellent and soon some added advantages became apparent. For since Lamprene checks the allergic flare-up that often comes with leprosy, it can be used continuously. Other drugs may have to be used intermittently, for the consequences of such allergies can be unpleasant. Although over the years Lamprene proved highly popular, it was expensive and patients on lengthy treatment showed changes in their skin color. Yet even where a large number of patients have been treated exclusively with Lamprene, some for more than ten years, only one case of resistance has ever been recorded.

With the third drug, rifampicin, the predictions of logic were totally fulfilled: it is highly effective against both tuberculosis and leprosy. Rifampicin is a potent antibiotic. Discovered in 1959 the red-colored fungus was first noticed in a wood in northern Italy, and got its name from a movie, *Rififi,* which was being filmed in that wood at that time. An Italian firm, Lepetit, first developed this antibiotic, then took it to Ciba-Geigy, and in 1966 Dr. Dennis Burley set up the first clinical trials in Great Britain, with a pioneer in tuberculosis treatment, Professor John Crofton. The patients responded so spectacularly that the drug rapidly became the first-line treatment for tuberculosis in many centers in Great Britain.

It was Dr. Colin McDougall at the Department of Dermatology at the Slade Hospital, Oxford, who first tried rifampicin against leprosy. From a number of centers there was a feeling that rifampicin might well prove useful. Clinicians made a rough guess what the dose should be, but no one knew how long to keep it up, or whether it should be administered every day for a week or two weeks or a month or a year. A small group of McDougall's leprosy patients were put on different periods and some, he now feels, received treatment for far too long. One group got the pill every day for a year, which, in retrospect, was totally unnecessary. But there were no adverse reactions and the regular routine monitoring of liver and blood function revealed no trouble at all. What McDougall does remember though, was the remarkable response of one patient, a mechanic working in a bus company at Reading, England. Originally from Pakistan, he had been regularly admitted to various hospitals around England because of a blocked-up nose, discharge, and bleeding, which had been going on for years. Quickly diagnosing him as having lepromatous leprosy, McDougall began administration of rifampicin immediately and forty-eight hours later the patient said: "Do you know, I can breathe through my nose for the first time since I came to this country, nine years ago." Up to that point he had thought that his trouble was caused by England's notoriously damp climate. After six months on rifampicin he went back to his job where, a healthy man, he is still repairing buses.

The response to rifampicin is extraordinarily quick, and the bacterial load in the body rapidly reduced to zero. In experimental animals the bacilli are killed within five to six *hours* and a patient treated with rifampicin will be excreting fragmented, dead bacilli within a matter of days. The effect is truly striking, because once the drug is absorbed it goes right through to the cells and interrupts the growth and division of the bacillus. Whereas other antibiotics, like penicillin and streptomycin, act only on cell walls, rifampicin gets to work right in the heart of the nucleus and so directly interferes with the genetic material of the bacillus.

Though the dream of all clinicians in tropical diseases is to have quick-acting therapeutic agents, the clinical problems leprologists face are of a different order or magnitude from those provoked by a few parasitic worms living in the body. For these small, highly specialized, mycobacilli are hidden deep, with a metabolism and growth so slow that they are formidably difficult to attack. They are exquisitely adapted to survive in the body's cells, and this is why even though rifampicin *is* fast-acting, treatment must go on for a long time.

Though new antileprosy agents are required and none are as yet on the horizon, the existing combination of the three drugs is nevertheless proving formidable. The new regimen, developed and recommended by WHO, involves the use of the three drugs in a well-defined pattern of administration. It aims to overcome a number of problems simultaneously, whether they be drug resistance or patient compliance. The recommended therapy for patients with the highly infectious, multibacillary leprosy is a self-administered (100 milligram) dose of dapsone and clofazimine daily, and a supervised, high dose (600 milligram) of rifampicin and clofazimine once a month.

There are three important points about this procedure. First, the probability of drug resistance with a single drug is a quantifiable measure; with two drugs resistance can be reduced by about a thousand; with three they are reduced to a thousand times a thousand, which is negligible. Second, the large, once monthly supervised dose of rifampicin and clofazimine covers several problems. If, either because of forgetfulness or because patients have lost their pills, the routine of the daily dose fails, the monthly supervised dose provides a considerable safeguard. A third problem relates to the general and very widespread use of rifampicin, which besides being an antileprosy drug is a most valuable antibiotic against not only tuberculosis but pneumonia and gonorrhea too. So valuable are the capsules now that in some countries they have become a currency in their own right, and patients are tempted to swipe a handful and hide them in their clothes. Having done so, they sell them on the black market, leaving their own leprosy untreated. In some areas in some countries, an appalling situation has arisen, with echoes of Graham Greene's *The Third Man*, the tale of black marketeers who sold dilute penicillin capsules with horrifying results in Vienna after World War II. Some people have been stealing the rifampicin, diluting it, making up the capsules again, and selling them at inflated prices. The consequences are terrible. Patients remain uncured; they develop allergic reactions to these small continuous doses; and the widespread use of these drugs once again will lead to drug resistance.

The new multidrug therapy has one specific objective then, to reduce the prevalence of leprosy progressively by hitting hard at the disease in those few people who can infect others, while at the same time still treating those with the less serious form. The whole schedule has now been formally adopted and is in effect in several countries. In one, Guyana, it was started early on with outstanding results. A British doctor in Guyana,

Pat Rose, was visited in 1981 by another Britisher who had just come from Geneva and had learned about the new recommendations. The visitor briefed her and very soon she started the six-month regimen for all paucibacillary patients in the country; it is now clear that she has treated virtually all of them. True, since neither the country nor its population is large, the total numbers weren't vast, but the principle established is critically significant. For having cured the simple cases Dr. Rose can now concentrate on the infectious, difficult forms and, it is believed, will soon complete total treatment of *all* categories of leprosy in Guyana. When this is done she may well have broken the chain of transmission of leprosy for the first time ever. She has an excellent chance of succeeding because she knows the leprosy population intimately, for unlike Nepal or India, the diseased population is confined to one place, the sugar plantations on the north coast.

Being in a committee room at WHO in Geneva is one thing and working in the crowded slums of Bombay, or the remote valleys of Bhutan, is quite another, and the success of any country's control program will be measured by the imagination and ingenuity with which each country adapts theory to suit its particular circumstances. Here it is clear why the role of the paramedical groups and the mobile clinics is so important in Nepal. If leprosy is controlled it will be because, backed up and encouraged by their government and the foreign missions, the Nepalese reeducate the Nepalese and themselves are willing to sacrifice time and energy to go to patients who cannot possibly travel to them. The aching muscles of the paramedics, their willingness to spend days away from home, their courage in the face of the social stigma that sometimes still adheres, their gentleness and the sensitivity with which they treat patients, talk to the villagers, and examine the small children will, in the end, be crucial – and, it is likely, successful – as I saw for myself at nine thousand feet. The patient there, Man Singh, was only one of many regularly visited. His therapy was sustained, he received a fresh supply of his daily drug, and was given his once-monthly, supervised dose of rifampicin, not just offered with a glass of water. The pill was placed on his tongue and water poured down his throat. The paramedics take no chances with rifampicin. What matter that water is sloshed all over his collar? The pill has got to go *down* and this is how the drug is routinely administered.

So if government plans go well and outside support is given so that the paramedical scheme, along with the mobile clinics and the referral centers, can be extended, then in probably no less than a decade leprosy could be effectively controlled in Nepal. Nevertheless some doubts remain.

Existing tools are not really sufficient, Narsappa "Sam" Samuel believes. There are several reasons why. We were talking with Dr. John Stanford, who had dropped in for a few days to review past and future work. The two were running a number of research projects together on the fundamental science of leprosy. We were strolling down the stone pathway to visit the Mycobacterial Research Laboratories, a long, two-storied building at the bottom of the campus, constructed on a gentle curve that commands the best views over the valley. Sam is intensely proud of these labs. For here, in the simplest of scientific settings, he has set up the most remarkable of scientific systems, maintaining colonies of infection-prone mice as competently as the most sophisticated scientific laboratory in the United States. Research colonies of "nude" mice, animals deliberately bred without a thymus gland so half their immune system is missing, are used everywhere to study infectious diseases, for they catch these easily. But so immunologically vulnerable are they that their cages must be maintained in the most aseptic of conditions and the technicians gowned and robed, as if working in a totally sterilized area in a hospital. Yet Sam maintains this system and gets good results using equipment discarded from U.S. laboratories. "We can use this," he said, "for six months, or more. We are happy to use it and we're not complaining."

We were down at an electron microscope, so arranged that as Sam manipulated a slide under the eyepiece, John and I could observe what he wished to describe. On the subject of whether the multidrug therapy gets rid of every single bacillus from the patient, Sam now explained: "I don't think this happens. Even after three years of treatment, multibacillary patients still have dead bacilli in their body, and there may be others still alive, that's very difficult for the drugs to deal with." John Stanford interjected:

What you've got to understand is that in dealing with either leprosy or tuberculosis the population of bacteria is really in two parts. There's the population actively multiplying in the diseased tissues, which is causing the infection, and there is no doubt that adequate drug therapy will kill off the vast majority of these organisms relatively quickly. But the reason why you can't then stop treatment is that there is a second population of bacilli in various parts of the body, which are either not multiplying at all, or are only doing so extremely slowly. They're not always in the lesions; they sometimes persist in the sites like the nerves where the tissues appear quite normal. Unfortunately if you stop treatment after you have just killed off the ones causing the disease, in one year or perhaps ten, these persisters will again begin to multiply. And this is where the tragedy of the immune status of the multibacillary patient becomes important, for their immune system can't "see" those persisters. This is the reason why we think that something extra – another therapy, immunotherapy – is going to be an essential adjunct to tomorrow's treatment of leprosy.

But to give the "something extra" one must know what is wrong with the immune system of these patients, and to know what is wrong, one must learn something of what normally goes on in a healthy body, when a bacillus invades. This John Stanford proceeded to explain.

Immune protection occurs in two ways, he reminded me. Sometimes chemical substances – antibodies – are produced that smother the functioning of invading bacteria. But protection also comes through cells that either eat up the invaders or produce substances to kill them. This process – cell-mediated immunity – is wonderful and complex, and involves a carefully regulated pattern of cooperative activity between the many different immune cells. It is by this process that an invasion of leprosy bacilli is tackled, and it is the lack of an effective cell-mediated immunity that causes the problem for multibacillary patients. In fact it is suspected that the range of responses to the leprosy bacilli reflects a parallel, underlying range of cell-mediated immunity in patients. In most of us our cellular response is superb; in paucibacillary patients it is not very good, and in multibacillary patients it is defective.

After the bacilli have penetrated the skin, the first cells to react are the macrophages, whose job it is literally to eat them up, assisted, activated, and perhaps even controlled by another special group of cells, the T-lymphocytes. Each macrophage advances remorselessly upon its victim and the bacillus is engulfed. Then as the bacillus disintegrates, some of its proteins appear on the surface of the macrophage and the presence of these triggers two further processes. First, other macrophages arrive to help, since, of course, there is always more than one invading bacillus. Second, some killer lymphocytes arrive and begin to proliferate many times. A complex chain of events now follows which ends with the destruction of all the invaders. It is this cellular activity that produces the first symptoms of leprosy on the skin surface, a white patch, the granuloma, that indicates an infectious invasion being repelled.

But this process must be controlled, for once all the invaders are killed, all action must cease. Now other T-cells, *suppressors,* call a halt by preventing the lymphocytes recognizing the surface molecules of the bacillus.

In the multibacillary patient, however, several things may be wrong, separately and together. First, the macrophage may itself be sick so the leprosy bacilli thrive inside. Second, the control mechanisms in the immune system may get completely out of hand, either because they are overpowered by invading bacilli or because something is defective in their mechanisms, or both. Then the suppressor cells that switch the system off predominate over the killer cells that help kill invaders. Scientists who hope to compensate for the defective immune system of a leprosy patient can try one of a number of things. They can find out what is wrong with the mechanisms of cell-mediated immunity; they can see whether any chemical substances are missing and, if so, try to supply them; they can try to retrain the macrophage to recognize the leprosy bacillus completely; finally, they can use vaccines to stimulate the immune system and enhance its actions. All approaches are being tried, and it is at this point that the work of a remarkable international network becomes critical. The existence of this network, which draws together both basic scientists and clinical leprologists from all over the world, is something quite new in the saga of the continuing struggle with leprosy.

In the past, leprosy was never a fashionable field, one whose attractions could be guaranteed to draw young researchers into a fascinating web of difficult problems. The brunt of the work was carried, clinically and scientifically, by a few saintly missionaries and a few devoted leprologists. The mainstream of research, which swept along cohorts of biologists, simply bypassed leprosy and its problems. But this is all changing fast, and the inherent challenges in leprosy are one reason why. One person whose career was redirected by leprosy, and who helped create the new network, is an internationally renowned immunologist, Dr. Barry Bloom, who is tackling the problem of the defective immune system.

When Bloom started in science he knew, as all scientists know, that the path to the top is notoriously straight and narrow and those who wish to garner the golden stars are well advised not to deviate. A distinguished graduate from that mecca of scientific research institutions, the Rockefeller University, his career was well under way and by 1967, he and his wife Irene had saved enough money for a house in Westchester in the New York suburbs. Suddenly they realized that they hadn't seen anything of the world and if they didn't go now they probably never would. So using their savings they went to India, Afghanistan, Pakistan, and Nepal. The next six weeks, Bloom says succinctly, "turned my whole life around."

When he first went to Asia the Third World was incomprehensible to him. But after their travels he not only became very receptive to different cultures, but also developed a strong personal obligation to find something useful that would come from his science. Until then his experience had been the same as that of most research scientists, limited, that is, to laboratory animals. "Nice little systems." he says, "in which no one ever gets sick and no one ever dies, for that's how you do science. But then we went to India and Nepal and saw lepers with no fingers and no faces, who were begging all over the place. I had nightmares, literally for weeks. So I came back and thought about them and soon found out that the whole disease is in my field."

This is, of course, true and soon Bloom was puzzling over the question: Why do the vast majority of people continually exposed never develop the disease? How do their defense systems recognize the bacillus and destroy it? Conversely, what is wrong with the immune systems of those four in every hundred people who succumb? Then, in 1972, not long after Bloom returned home from his trip to Asia, WHO convened a meeting in Delhi on the immunology of leprosy organized by Dr. Howard Goodman, the "Sol Hurok of international health," Bloom calls him, the head of WHO's Immunology Unit and a scientific impresario. Having a deep conviction that immunology lay at the core of the leprosy problem, Goodman called together a group of people, some of whom, "while not perhaps even knowing what a Third World disease was," commented Bloom, "were doing good immunology." It was a unique occasion, for work on leprosy was still more or less the sole property of a few clinical leprologists.

Bloom recalls the scientific meeting as one of the most extraordinary events of his life.

There were I think six people who counted and three of us knew nothing whatever about leprosy – Tony Allison, and Tore Godal, the Norwegian, – and while, sure, I had seen people with no fingers or noses, I actually knew nothing about the disease at all. The three other people were classical, old-time leprologists and the meeting was at levels of lack of communication like I have never seen before. But it was very exciting because we had the questions and they had the answers. So we sat these guys down who, at that time, didn't know a T-lymphocyte from an antibody and said, "What is this?, What is that?" And they would tell us about the patients and whether their white cell counts were going up or down. Then we sat down and wrote a technical bulletin.

The real hero is Tore Godal. He was the catalyst who got the network off and running, the guy who glued this odd, disparate collection of people together. The result was that we formulated some hypotheses and devised protocols to test all the immunology potentials of leprosy patients. The Norwegian government was sufficiently impressed to give us $700,000 each year, and with this we started IMLEP, which is WHO's scientific working group in the immunology of leprosy. We realized very quickly that the patients were in one place and the scientists in another – in fact everybody was all over the place and nobody could do the whole job. So we shared out the work. Now this is something which has not been notably successful in science before and many scientists will tell you that it cannot be done. But they are wrong. Though some people still argue that an international organization like WHO cannot get anything done, for people bicker and fight and all too often the money is allocated according to a country's politics, it didn't work out like that for us and it doesn't work out like that for most of the WHO tropical disease programs.

Of the activities now supported, research into the immunology of leprosy was one; another was the making of a leprosy vaccine. By 1984, twelve years after that initial meeting in Delhi, both objectives had been met. The medical world has a far better idea of what is wrong with, and how to go about compensating for, the defective immune systems of those multibacillary patients, and it has a vaccine.

First, the immune defects: wherever and whatever, it is now clear that they are not in the macrophage, the cell that first eats up the leprosy bacilli, because they continue to respond against an invasion of the mycobacilli of tuberculosis. But the leprosy bacillus somehow manages to hoodwink the cells of the immune system. It seems to do so, by sending trigger signals to those suppressor cells that *stop* the process whereby the macrophages digest the bacilli. Whereas in paucibacillary leprosy the macrophages do manage to destroy most of the leprosy organisms, in multibacillary leprosy they do not, so now the bacilli multipy inside *them* just as successfully as they do outside.

In an elegantly designed series of experiments Barry Bloom and his colleagues at the Albert Einstein School of Medicine in the Bronx, New York, have unraveled a possible mechanism for the signals that the hoodwinking bacilli transmit. Like many signals in the body, this is biochemical: a complicated molecule on the surface of the bacillus is formed of one fatty part with three sugar "partners" and the sugar part is the crucial element. When this "signal," this molecule, is added to a culture of white blood cells from multibacillary patients, the immune response is damped down and so, too, is the activity of those other immune cells that normally stimulate the macrophages into further defensive action. Bloom believes this surface molecule is quite specific to the leprosy bacilli, evidence of the exquisite evolutionary adaptiveness of the organism. For it evolved to "mimic" the suppressor cells by triggering their functional effect and so ensuring that the leprosy bacilli evade the net of immune surveillance.

The first answer to the question, what is unusual, immunologically speaking, in the severe form of leprosy, is a property peculiar to the bacillus. By contrast, the Norwegian Tore Godal, working with the Ethiopians in the Armauer Hansen Institute in Addis Ababa, has demonstrated that another thing wrong is peculiar to the immune system of those patients: one vital protein is missing from the chain of defense reactions. This substance, interleukin II, is produced in a normal immune response and both activates the macrophage and stimulates the proliferation of other white cells. Multibacillary patients do not appear to be making it; but once again, if it is added to a culture of their immune cells, the activating function is restored.

Dr. Naida Nogueira, a Brazilian at New York University, has also approached the problem from a similar tack. Working on the same hypothesis – that the defective immune system lacked substances that trigger the macrophages – she showed that yet another substance was crucial, *gamma interferon,* and that the difference between paucibacillary and multibacillary patients was that the latter never produced this protein. Now she asked: Do they lack the capacity to make gamma interferon at all, or has something else failed in the whole complicated chain? Here the work of Godal merged with hers to give a neat picture of what is happening. Some cells make chemical messengers to communicate between those cells, macrophages, which eat up foreign matter, and those lymphocytes, that make antibodies, which cooperate together to mount a defense. It is interleukin II that "tells" all these cells to get the act together. The links in the chain are as follows. Multibacillary patients are missing interleukin II, the substance which, when a foreign agent appears in the blood, tells the macrophages to make another substance, gamma interferon. This substance in its turn triggers the activity of other macrophages, and this leads to the mobilization of the crucial killer lymphocytes, which proliferate a hundredfold. Happily, all this work may lead directly to therapy, for it suggests what pharmaceutical substances might one day be used to remedy the immune defect in these leprosy patients.

Finally there is John Stanford's approach to the problem, one that is, quite literally, more earthy. Whereas Bloom and the immunologists are asking what happens between the macrophage and other immune cells, he is asking questions about what the bacilli are doing to the macrophage. One group looks at the problem from the stance of infection, the other from the stance of immune response to that infection. Since he is confident that his ideas are right but believes, too, that Drs. Bloom, Godal, and Nogueira are also probably right, John Stanford suspects that eventually they are all going to come to arrive at the same point.

He expounded this on the green terraced lawn of the Samuels' house in Nepal, against the backcloth of a small golden valley from which the wooded green hills rose steeply some five miles away. With his enormous frame, great red beard, and shock of red hair, he looked like a biblical prophet who wanders in the wilderness, and wander he does. He is a game hunter and he has been to many remote areas; the organisms he captures are not big game but small – bacteria. I was asking him how he could be so confident that I wouldn't get leprosy during my stay in Nepal, even though I would be challenged with the bacilli many times. What was going to protect me, he answered, was basically my English background and by this he didn't mean where I went to school. He was talking about the environment that I had made during my life – the organisms and substances I have met and to which my own immune system had learned to respond.

Look at that valley behind us. It contains a greater collection of mycobacteria than anywhere else in the whole world, and these people are meeting these bacilli *every* day. When I was in Uganda thirteen years ago, I looked at the distribution of three mycobacterial diseases and I realized that they could be related to observable geographic differences. Though it wasn't by any means entirely my idea, I suspected that the most obvious thing which could influence this would be that the organisms causing the diseases were also distributed geographically. So wherever we went, we took samples of mud, water, grass, to see whether there were mycobacteria common in all the samples, or if there weren't, and if this related to the spread of diseases. Well it did, and this started me off looking at all forty species of mycobacteria, to see how they relate not only to disease they provoke, but to the fact that some people can mount a defense and others can't.

When John Stanford first came to Anandaban in 1979 he wanted to know what other mycobacteria, beside those responsible for leprosy and tuberculosis, were present. In the surrounding valley he found *every* one of the forty species. He took samples from the soil, scrapings from the standpipes, drops from the pools, smears from the stone depressions. Under his microscope he saw mycobacteria, very dark red rods sitting on top of brown dirt. Every pot filled from the tap, or every vessel dipped in the pool, contained the whole range of bacilli and people met them every time they drank or washed. Thus the beautiful valley below Anandaban conceals hidden dangers, and the Nepalese meet many more such bacilli than the Eskimos in the Arctic or the nomads in the Sahara.

So far as the capacity to mount an effective defense against mycobacterial disease is concerned, Stanford believes that you're in trouble if you meet too few bacilli and you're in trouble if you meet too many. The Eskimos are rarely in trouble because where they live few bacilli are around. Conversely an Eskimo meeting a missionary with infectious tuberculosis would be felled by the disease, since his immune system had never met the infection before. On the other hand, Indians, Africans, or people in Nepal meet so many bacilli that their immune systems rapidly become overloaded and may be even in a state of permanent suppression. Such a possibility has only been recognized over the last few years. This is what John Stanford believes is happening to people in the valley behind Anandaban. The people constantly receive infections through the mouth, and the overload eventually leads to permanent suppression of their immune systems. But, as he quickly added, this is only today's hypothesis and by tomorrow it might have changed.

Thus, whereas Bloom thinks that a protein on the surface of the leprosy bacillus triggers the suppression of immunity, Stanford believes that this is caused by a mixed bacillary overload. As might be expected, their differing ideas are reflected in the vaccines – the second target of the network's research – they are providing.

The vaccine that Stanford and Sam use is made from a harmless bacillus taken from the roots of a muddy grass plant, growing in a Ugandan lake. All forty species of mycobacteria share some common surface molecules, called antigens, that trigger immune protection. So the two researchers have made a preparation from this organism, which when injected presents someone with a bundle of these protective antigens. In one trial the local schoolchildren have been vaccinated with this alone, or with this and the antitubercular vaccine BCG, with one group remaining as controls. In addition they tried to find those children who have the characteristic defect in their immune system and vaccinate them *before* they contracted leprosy. The first signs are hopeful; an increasing number of children are responding to their vaccine in ways which shows that their immunity to leprosy is increasing.

At the same time Sam is using the vaccine as an immunotherapy to plug the gap he mentioned earlier, to try, that is, to improve the immune status of those multibacillary patients who, though they can be well treated by drugs, are in danger of relapsing. These patients continue to receive multidrug therapy but also receive injections of vaccine plus BCG, at regular intervals. Now he is finding that not only are *all* the bacilli disappearing but that the patients are eliminating the dead ones faster. Clinically they are much better and so, too, is their immune response. Thus, whether it is a patient with multibacillary leprosy, or a healthy child found to be at risk from it, both are being "taught" to recognize the antigens associated with a protective immunity.

The vaccine Barry Bloom and other immunologists in the IMLEP network wanted to try would come from the leprosy bacilli themselves.

But whereas Stanford and Samuel get all the vaccine they want by treating soil samples, the IMLEP group was faced with the unwelcome fact that the leprosy bacillus will not grow in culture. What then could they possibly use as a factory? Of all the possible candidates the nine-banded armadillo surely must be the most unlikely, but this actually is the animal they use, for it turns out to be a lumbering agar dish. If an armadillo catches leprosy, it cultures the bacilli profusely. It was pure luck that this animal became involved. Dr. Eleanor E. Storrs, a biologist, happened to go to several leprosy conferences with her husband, a specialist on leprosy drugs, and repeatedly heard scientists moan about how refractory the bacillus was to cultivate and how it liked cool places. So one day she simply put up her hand and said, "Why not try my armadillos?" explaining that their body temperature is some five degrees lower than most other animals.

In 1970 the chief of the Laboratory Research at the National Hansen's Disease Center in Louisiana was persuaded to inoculate armadillos. It worked like a dream: they came down with human leprosy and were soon swarming with bacilli. They have to be regularly captured in the wild because they will not reproduce in captivity. Intriguingly they react to leprosy in the same way as humans; only half succumb, so the other half are released. To their considerable surprise, the first job of Barry Bloom and his colleagues in WHO's special leprosy program was to support people who had the know-how to keep colonies of captive armadillos happy. Each 4.5 kilogram of sick armadillo yields nearly 250 grams of infected tissue, which contain as many as one million million bacilli per gram. "If you make certain assumptions," says Bloom dreamily, "between fifty and five hundred armadillos might provide vaccine for the whole world."

Someone next had to extract pure bacilli from the messy infected tissues of the first armadillos auditioned for this role, and this is where the network of international scientists with special individual skills is called into play. The spleen and liver tissues are packed in solid carbon dioxide, kept at minus 70 degrees Fahrenheit and air-freighted to the Laboratory for Leprosy and Mycobacterial Research at the National Institutes for Medical Research at Mill Hill, London. It was a lanky biochemist in his mid-thirties, Philip Draper, and Dick Rees, then head of the Laboratory, who devised the successful technique. It took them five years, some luck, a small amount of money, and an enormous amount of work. But Bloom calls Draper "a wizard" for given a "terrible mess" and told to produce undamaged bacilli, he does. Draper volunteers that the duration of the process depends on how organized he is. It was possible to start with messy tissue in the morning and have a suspension of pure bacillus by teatime, but generally he spreads the operation over two days because there's really no need to hurry and that way it's less of a strain.

Philip Draper now packs the pure bacilli into small phials to be air-freighted to Bloom at Albert Einstein College of Medicine in New York City, to Thomas Buchanan at the U.S. Public Health Service Hospital in Seattle, to Morten Harboe at the National Hospital at the University of Oslo, Norway; other samples go to Ethiopia, to France, and to Australia, for the next task is to see whether the material is of any use, immunologically speaking. Is it carrying useful antigens and will it provoke in mice those effective immune reactions? Buchanan looks for possible defects in the suspensions; Harboe identifies the crucial surface molecules and makes antibodies against them; in Louisiana, Kirschheimer vaccinates more armadillos with his lot while Bloom in New York tests the degree of immune response in laboratory animals. To all participants' delight, the dead bacilli turned out to be immunologically most potent.

By January 1981 all was ready for safety trials and the Wellcome drug company in England was granted a license to produce the IMLEP vaccine for human use. The United States was chosen for the trial for it had neither tuberculosis nor leprosy vaccination, nor many lepers, so nothing would complicate the testing. The hardest part was finding a population settled enough to be followed for years. The leprosy bacillus doubles every twelve to twenty-two days; nothing in the world grows slower. Since nothing comes on fast, nothing goes away quickly, and this has a bearing on the second thing scientists have to know: how long does protection last? Will one shot do or will boosters be necessary? Subjects would have to be found who were traceable, so that their immune response could be tested every two years, five years, perhaps even *ten* years. Barry Bloom thinks that medical students, the usual volunteers, are unsuitable for this very reason, and the laboratories at the National Institutes of Health, or the Center for Disease Control, with their relatively permanent staffs, will be the places to tap.

Clinical safety trials actually began in May 1982 in Norway and the United Kingdom too, besides North America. There were two scientific and political reasons for this wide choice besides the fact that the IMLEP network wanted to study the vaccine clean, without the intervention of major disease complications or prior exposure to leprosy. But the second reason highlights what can be an acute political dilemma. People in the Third World are very sensitive to the fact that many drug protocols are first tried out on them. The IMLEP Committee wanted the vaccine to be tested in volunteers from Europe and America so no question of Third World guinea pig populations could arise. The first phase of the trial should reveal an appropriate dose and then a second group of people will be vaccinated, to be monitored for a decade. Further trials will then be conducted in the developing world to test the actual efficacy of the vaccine.

There are still several problems however, one of which can be stated quite simply: If nature has already separated out those 96 percent of people with immunity to leprosy from those remaining who cannot mount an immune response, why should we expect a vaccine to work at all, seeing that all it does is merely perform "unnaturally" what nature does spontaneously? How can we hope to do what nature herself does not? This argument applies equally to any vaccine, whether made from other mycobacteria or from the leprosy bacilli, and there is a tremendous debate as to whether or not a vaccine will be of any use. But preliminary trials in Venezuela and in Nepal indicate that it really does work though no one really understands why.

Despite debate over who should receive these vaccines, there is general agreement that the situation is not like polio, smallpox, or hepatitis B. Scientists will not just inject the vaccine into millions of people who will then be protected against leprosy. In any case since the majority of people cope easily with a challenge from leprosy, mass vaccination would be a ridiculous waste of time and resources. So the use of the vaccine will be focused primarily on the walking cultures of bacilli, those silent multibacillary patients: the first task will be to use the vaccine – as Sam and John Stanford use theirs – as an adjunct to drug treatment, and help both clear infection and build up an immunological memory.

Sam showed me three people who had been treated this way. One had mild leprosy, one had no disease but was in close contact with those who had, and one had a severe form of multibacillary disease. All were given a course of vaccination with BCG added, and some weeks later their immune response was measured with a skin biopsy. Both the young man and the young girl with no previous immunity were now showing a positive reaction, but most remarkable of all was the response of the severely diseased patient. His bacilli were actively degrading and even more important, the activity of his macrophages had been greatly stimulated and a major immunological response mounted. These results parallel those of Dr. Convit, in Venezuela, who has been giving similar immunotherapy to leprosy patients for a long time now, with great success. Many scientists find these results exciting but, again, extremely surprising. Dr. Dick Rees of Mill Hill explains why:

The results really amaze us. We were astonished that Dr. Convit hasn't run into tremendous adverse, allergic reactions when giving repeated doses of the vaccine. We were also very surprised, because patients with multibacillary leprosy have already huge numbers of the bacilli inside them. Indeed by the time the disease appears they probably even have an allergy to the bacillus. So to give them yet more bacilli in a vaccine? We felt that this couldn't possibly do anything. Perhaps it is the addition of the BCG, acting as an enhancer. But very likely the process is even more cunning. Possibly the BCG is turning something on in the lymphocytes that somehow allows the leprosy bacilli to show their antigenic molecules.

And, perhaps the "something" being turned on is one of the substances that the immunologists have discovered to be missing. Dr. Naida Nogueira planned to visit Anandaban and hoped to monitor immunologically the patients who are responding to their vaccine preparations. She wants to see whether the effect of the vaccine indeed induces the lymphocytes to make gamma interferon, the substance that provokes the macrophages into doing their proper job. If it does, then John Stanford's prediction will be borne out, the wheel will have come full circle, and the approaches of the bacteriologists and immunologists will finally merge.

For Ram Baradur Lama, alone in the jungle for eleven years, all these exciting results have come too late. But the cured Shanta Maya, hopping about on her one leg, and Bhim Prasad, guiding his plough with a functioning hand, and Goma Bandari, delicately selecting wheat grains with working fingers under the critical eye of her mother-in-law, and Rameysh, the clown, somersaulting in the ring, can hope: perhaps they themselves really are the last generation of leprosy patients and their children will be free.

But perhaps they will not. For one must weigh the strength of the medical armamentarium against the problems of applying effective medical solutions. While on the one hand, there is no reason at all why their children should *not* be free, sadly, it is most unlikely that they will, and there are various reasons why.

One solution to leprosy was always breathtakingly simple but appallingly difficult to apply, namely economic development. Look back four hundred years to medieval Europe and we see that suddenly the disease apparently vanished. But it wasn't sudden at all. At the end of the Middle Ages there was still a great deal of leprosy in Europe and it took over two hundred years before a significant decrease occurred, and still we don't know what were the factors responsible. John Stanford would say a level of cleanliness that came when we began to place barriers between us and the earth, such as floors in our houses and shoes on our feet. Others say more frequent washing of people and more frequent changes of clothes; others a higher level of general health and better resistance resulting from better socioeconomic conditions, where these involved a number of factors, from less overcrowding to better food. Nor is it really strictly correct to say that leprosy has vanished from Europe, because where the appalling conditions recur, so too does leprosy. A vicious circle is quickly set up, where malnutrition and insanitation provoke general states of debilitation which, in turn, lower resistance and provoke more disease, which burdens the immune system.

Nevertheless, the gradual disappearance of leprosy from Europe was a genuine phenomenon, so improving living and general economic conditions in the Third World should have the same effect. But given present realities, and the wide indifference to the living conditions of the rural poor, we must ask whether we prefer to have an aggressive attitude to leprosy now, or leave things to improve on their own, or hope for development, in which case progress will be painfully slow. Both WHO and most governments are realists and know that they must aim to reduce the global load of infection *now,* by concentrating the drug regimen on multibacillary patients and so reduce the amount of leprosy around.

But several things are going to be required to achieve even *this.* Adequate control depends on drugs and though the new combinations are far more effective and, as Pat Rose's example in Guyana shows, can bring about dramatic changes, they are also still too expensive. WHO estimates that it would cost approximately thirty dollars per year to treat a multibacillary patient with multidrug therapy; with dapsone alone the cost was only two dollars. And though potential vaccines are in clinical trial, these will not be cheap to develop or to administer, and will take perhaps twenty years to prove their worth. This may equally be true of whatever drugs result from the work of immunologists. If interferons are the therapeutic keys to immunological success here, then we *are* in a difficulty, for the human body produces them only in very small quantity and they are correspondingly expensive to produce.

But money isn't the real problem. Even supplying all the drugs free of charge would be a futile gesture without the proper infrastructure to deliver them. The problem has now become less a question of basic science than of mechanisms of delivery and commitment. Unfortunately, part of the pattern in a developing country is that either there is no infrastructure for health or a totally inadequate one. For effective leprosy control a health system must detect the maximum number of patients as early as possible and treat them appropriately as quickly as possible. And though the special problems of such varied countries as Nepal, India, Ethiopia, Guyana, and the Philippines will dictate different forms of health systems, they share some common needs for leprosy control. These include an administration, commitment, personnel, and finance, of an order of focused magnitude that has *never* been attempted before in leprosy. No longer can the situation be handled by idealistic and medically qualified missionaries, working in remote stations isolated from the general community. A veritable army of people will be needed, with training in leprosy detection and control, and all this means a major change in local government policy.

Certainly there are many governments which over the past decade have given a very high priority to leprosy. India is one, so too is Ethiopia. But in general leprosy has been placed on the ladder of health care many times lower than malaria or the more communicable diseases. Giving priority to leprosy entails an active decision and certainly finances allocated are slowly increasing. But once again as with drugs, and money, so too with intentions: there is a big gap between means and will.

One crucial aspect in this is a corresponding lack of interest in the medical profession. Leprosy control is considered a low-level assignment and doctors prefer to concentrate on more fashionable specialities. Leprosy never provided a good career with which to earn money or gain status, and within the medical profession there is still great reluctance to deal with leprosy patients. The prejudice that exists among the patients' families and the communities, exists here also. Paramedics, too, in many countries have showed they don't like to work in leprosy; Dr. Adiga often spoke of the social sacrifices they made and how the government of Nepal tries to compensate for these. So a second vicious circle is quickly set up. When a government gives high priority to leprosy, the action has to extend to the medical schools. A survey made in India, for example, a few years back, revealed that students were taught about leprosy on average for only four and a half hours of their entire six years' training, even though there are more leprosy victims in India than anywhere else on earth. By contrast, in Ethiopia, where for many years there has been a strong commitment both to leprosy control and basic research, all medical students are required to work in the leprosy hospital and research laboratories in Addis Ababa for at least three months.

Still Indira Gandhi often spoke of eradicating leprosy in India by the year 2000. Nepal hopes to control it by 1990. The Chinese also have decided that leprosy will be eradicated by the year 2000; there the disease has already declined from half a million in 1949 to approximately 200,000 people in 1983, a drop attributed to a combination of improved living standards and new drug treatments aggressively applied. When asked whether these were achievable targets, the director of WHO's Leprosy Unit, Dr. Sansarricq, replies:

Well, first you have to make a definition of what eradication is. If eradication is a level of transmission of leprosy in which only occasional cases of the disease occur, perhaps one could do it. With modern drug therapy we could get the problem down to a situation where we would be having to deal with only 10 or at the very most 20 percent of the patients we had ten years ago. But this method only works when detection and treatment are run in parallel in very precise ways and with total coverage.

But the year 2000 is really very near and from the epidemiological point of view, there is no great hope that the multidrug therapy will break the transmission of the disease totally. Because, at present, when one is clinically able to detect a multibacillary patient, one has to assume that he has already spread the disease around, and given its long incubation new cases will be appearing in five or ten years. So while there has been a big decrease in the total number of cases there has been practically no decrease in the proportion of new ones appearing each year. And *that* is the reason why we need that vaccine. If we can use it to identify people at risk, or people with early disease and then treat, we will, in ten years, have both prevented the deformities and got rid of most patients. So in the end, if it proves not possible to do more while waiting for a development, I would consider that what we would have achieved would be very positive, even if those who are still patients are more difficult to cure than those who already have been cured.

When Bloom decided to focus his research on leprosy, he did so because it provided him (and, he insists, the rest of us) with a number of challenges. "Leprosy is not just a medical condition," he believes. "It is a disease of the body, of the mind, and of society. It presents an extraordinary, and perhaps unique, challenge of trying to do something. Twelve million people a year are estimated to have leprosy; their lives are ruined. So if with the limited expertise one has been trained to have, one sees an opportunity to make a contribution for ten million, two million, one million or just one person, this strikes me as an obligation." It is *our* obligation too. There is something very paradoxical about leprosy: we think it horrible but actually have used it as a great spiritual convenience.

Leprosy has always been a cause with its own unique appeal. At one and the same time we felt good because we were helping its victims with our charity, yet we rationalized our remoteness because so dreadful were the deformities that only saints could be involved. So with cash we ordinary mortals absolved ourselves from direct involvement. But in truth our attitudes are not much further advanced than those of the elderly people in the village who threw Ram Baradur out into the jungle. Still we create outcasts. Recently a radio broadcast in San Francisco revealed that in California there were two hundred patients reporting leprosy, expatriates from Vietnam or recent immigrants. The pressure at once generated to stop immigration of Vietnamese refugees became overwhelming. Barry Bloom himself was directly exposed to the unique stigma that still prevails, from a most unexpected source. Medical students are usually most willing volunteers for long-term safety trials on new vaccines, and without their help drug therapy would be light years behind. Recently, Bloom gave a lecture about the new, very *dead*, inactive and quite safe, leprosy vaccine to the medical students of his own college, Albert Einstein, and asked for volunteers to join the first preliminary safety trials. Usually he gets a massive response, but now only one student came forward. Another example concerns research. About twenty-five years ago Dr. James Hirsch's laboratory at Rockefeller University, New York, wanted to study the macrophages of leprosy patients for the light they rightly suspected they might throw on basic immunological processes. But it was decided that the university probably could not withstand the outcry that might arise if leprosy patients were known to be in the vicinity of the fashionable Upper East side of Manhattan. Two years ago however, leprosy patients from Staten Island began to be admitted on a once-a-week outpatient basis to the Rockefeller University Hospital, for Dr. Zanvill Cohen's laboratory, a linear intellectual descendant of Jim Hirsch's, has begun to study the problem that was articulated so many years back. Still some of the nurses expressed grave disquiet.

So the answer to the question, what prevents us from controlling leprosy worldwide, is still fear and indifference – an indifference that extends to many groups. It extends to governments in the developing world who pay mere lip service to the disease problems of their rural poor. It extends to those in the developed world who are reluctant to help or who will not believe that a society cannot pull itself up by its bootstraps if it doesn't have any boots. And the indifference extends to that mass of scientists who flock to the frontiers of molecular biology because their profession has no career structure and few rewards to encourage them in such unfashionable fields. Leprosy itself remains the outcast, presenting a stark gap between what is possible to achieve and what is likely to happen. So when one considers the actions needed in terms of realities present, the truthful and sober assessment must be pessimistic. Yet not only is it possible that those happy, smiling children of Nepal could see leprosy controlled, it is practical too, and it could be done with finances that, on a global scale, are minuscule.

Why should anyone devote time to leprosy and its patients when, compared to diseases like malaria, the numbers are so small? Are there surely not many more serious problems? And isn't the problem, anyway, light years away from the concerns of most medical researchers? My devil's advocate questions elicited a passionate response from Barry Bloom:

There are a number of reasons. The main one is because you can do something: for the first time since earliest recorded history we have the potential for eliminating this disease. There is a second reason: it is a minor disease if one only asks the question how many people have it? But it is a major one if you ask, what does it do to their lives? Patients who have very severe deformities still face a taboo beyond belief. They are fit to be beggars but nothing else, and this is not helping themselves or the countries in which they live. Third, we have a moral obligation. We have the most sophisticated biomedical establishment in the world in the United States. You can ask the people in Uganda and Upper Volta and Nepal to do a lot of things for themselves, but right now you can't ask them to make vaccines to cure their own diseases. But with very limited cost we can help – and for a lot less than we spend on guns. The whole tropical disease program at WHO, the whole shooting match for the control and research into six major tropical diseases, is less than the price of *one* single F18 jet fighter plane.

There are further reasons. I said we should study leprosy because we can *do* something and I also say we should study leprosy because we can *learn* something and not just about leprosy. You never know where knowledge is going to come from. I am always reminded of the team at Rockefeller University led by Avery in the early 1940s. Their job was pedestrian – studying pneumococcal bacilli to try and make a vaccine against pneumococcal pneumonia, the predominant medical problem during the Second World War. Well, along the way, they stumbled on the fact that a peculiar set of molecules, called DNA, carries inheritance. Curiously enough, they never made a vaccine for pneumococcal pneumonia, but they laid the scientific base for all the work on the gene that goes on in the world today.

Now I can show you something of what we are going to learn as we study leprosy. I believe that the mechanism by which people with multiple sclerosis damage their brains and nerves, resembles, at least histologically speaking, the way that paucibacillary leprosy patients damage their nerves. We have even set up an experimental animal model for this. We can place any foreign protein near myelinated nerves and show that the immune response to it, at that site, either strips off the myelinated sheath of the nerves or actually kills them. Leprosy does this, too. There are many diseases which result in an inflammatory stripping of the nerves and leprosy is one way of getting at the problem.

We can also learn something fundamental about immunological tolerance. Whereas our immune cells recognize and destroy foreign invaders they do not, except in very rare cases, recognize and destroy our own tissues. Now some people with leprosy don't recognize the bacillus either and by any immunological criteria whatever, the immune cells are not responding at all. So from an immunologist's point of view such patients demonstrate the truly fundamental phenomenon of *immunological tolerance,* and as such provide us with an absolute gold mine for research. It's the only system I know of in man in which we can get at that problem, and when we have cracked this, it will shed light on how it is also that some people fail to recognize their own cancers, for something similar is going on in cancer.* So parenthetically this work takes us from the rear end of science, which is leprosy, to the very forefront: human immunology.

But finally, in working with people in developing countries, we keep the spirit of questioning alive. That's what scientific work and scientific inquiry do and in my judgment the intellectual tradition of science has as much impact on the development of a country as material aid. Even Ethiopia's socialist revolutionary government, with its direction toward applied research, knows that in some way they need science there as a matter of keeping the country intellectually honest. So one of the greatest subversions to a totalitarian régime is the spirit of science because it is the spirit of free inquiry.

For whatever reason – moral imperative, nagging conscience, basic research, direct self-interest, or saintly devotion – leprosy continues to provide us with a singular index to our own attitudes. Bloom spends a lot of time on such extrascientific matters and some say his career has suffered. But being the kind of man he is, that visit to the Indian subcontinent inevitably provoked a change of ambition and though he may have paid a price for this he is intensely proud, as others are too, of the remarkable international network that now exists.

John Stanford sees the network as absolutely essential for the problems of the developing world:

In the future, we are going to need a continuation of this interchange between sophisticated laboratories and the field. The few examples like Anandaban, which have their own research laboratories, are of the very greatest benefit, because although they will never be able to do the most sophisticated and up-to-date things that are being done in Europe and in America, they are able to take the spin-offs and apply them in the field. So the useful tests developed overseas can be applied directly to leprosy patients, and their validity tested in a way which fits in with the patient's well-being. Only in a place like Nepal could the field studies be done

* It was announced in November, 1984 that the crucial protein, interleukin II, has also been successfully used against certain tumors. When injected into the tumor, the mass shrinks and the macrophages and lymphocytes, hitherto absent from the site, come in and start their work.

which could lead to the development of a successful vaccine. Although in the West we can carry out pilot experiments, either with laboratory animals or by using comparable diseases like tuberculosis, it requires a situation like this, where there is a real problem with leprosy, before we can measure whether the methods we are developing are really going to be of any use.

"There is nothing else like this network," said Dr. Dick Rees, in his turn. He had just retired from the Medical Research Council's leprosy laboratory at Mill Hill.

This is a magnificent internationally collaborative program and I have never yet before been on a steering or a planning committee run entirely by scientists. Usually they don't work because scientists fall out with each other or some of them decide to go off by themselves. We have stood very well together, we have shared out each problem, we all do our special parts, and we remain entirely open.

Such openness, though, exacts its price in the present competitive world of science, and other scientists looking at the program are cynical. It is open, they say, only because interest in leprosy is still so small. But just wait until the topic gets really hot and the scent of Nobel prizes is in the air, then watch the group fall apart. It's a moot point but most of the people in the network can't do science any other way. Bloom is sufficiently human, his wife admits, to be rueful when he considers the rewards and status of others, yet still they remain open. He, and his colleagues, present *all* their data at meetings and thus, periodically, must watch themselves being "scooped." But Bloom is philosophical and takes a long-term point of view:

Look, when you are a school kid, you think if you do good work you will get straight A's throughout your scientific career and all gold stars. Then you start in the lab on your problems and you find that you fail 99.9 percent of the time. So when you succeed and still someone has beat you by three weeks, then you are very ready to kill yourself. It is a funny way to make a living.

My disillusionment came early and this perhaps explains my commitment to team work. Once I really thought that, to a large extent, science was an area where individuals change the way of thinking about things and make an enormous contribution. But that's not the stuff of science and I learned very quickly that my uniqueness, which I treasured and believed in, is *not* so unique. There are lots of smart people out there and if I don't do it today somebody else is going to do it tomorrow.

So the disillusionment had to do with the twofold aspects one has to come to terms with. When you accept the role of the individual, then you redefine the rules and become a cooperative member in a cooperative group. Now the unique thing about our leprosy network is this: if you don't have that burning need to be the world's most famous and greatest and most wonderful scientist, which is part of the present problem in science, then you get your "jollies" from other things. One is to take on a complicated problem and work with, instead of against, other people. That, for me, is the most rewarding thing that's going. In contrast to what most people see or write [about science], whether overtly, consciously, or not – that science is people competing with each other – I see science as a cooperative enterprise. So why not come out and say, "It *is* a cooperative enterprise and I will send my stuff to the best guy so he can do something with it?" So any cell we have ever had, any virus we meet, we will give away. Sure those bastards will screw us all over with grants and do the work smarter and better, but that's the way it is. I don't think there is any *one* way to do science, and it grieves me to have to admit that some of the people who are the most secretive, competitive, and aggressive, do the best science. But the only way *I* can do science is as a societal activity, for one doesn't work in a desert island.

In a disease where the patients are in one country, the expertise on the bacilli in another, the biochemists in a third, the immunologists in a fourth, the pharmacists in a fifth, and the epidemiologists somewhere else, the only way to tackle a major problem is to establish a network and hang together as a team.

I'll show you the epigraph to a paper I wrote in 1971, even before I ever got deeply involved with leprosy. I'm an epigraph freak and that's my epigraph.

The epigraph read:

"Only connect."

E. M. Forster, *Howard's End*

A small, black-bearded Indian argues intently with a large, red-bearded Englishman, then drives to Kathmandu to place a telephone call to a restless, spectacled American. Sam and John decide they need some serum samples and Barry will have them flown over. Meantime a Venezuelan clinician is injecting some of his patients with a vaccine preparation derived from the work of a London biochemist, and assessed by a Norwegian immunologist, while a veterinarian in Louisiana wonders how many more armadillos he will be releasing back to the wild next week. And a young Indian surgeon writes a letter to a middle-aged science writer to say she's just clocked up another first. She has just done her first face lift on a badly deformed patient and it has gone very well.

What an odd, wonderful, paradoxical lot we humans are, I thought, as I read Susie's letter. The problems of the world's oldest and most horrifying disease, from whose victims most of us have backed away in revulsion, have generated the most remarkable cooperative network in science and the connections are holding firm.

5
The Last Wild Virus

All the business of war, and indeed all the business of life, is to endeavour to find out what you don't know by what you do; that's what I call, "Guessing what was at the other side of the hill."

It has been a damned serious business — the nearest run thing you ever saw in your life.

The Duke of Wellington on Waterloo,
Croker Papers (1885), Vol. III, p. 276

There presently exists a very small and exclusive international association and although there are no officers, annual dinners, headquarters, tax-deductible subscriptions, or conferences, the members insist that they are incredibly privileged. The chances of meeting a member are remote for, in numbers just over seven hundred, they are scattered over the face of the earth – from the Philippines to Senegal, from Thailand to Colombia – in refugee camps or in health organizations. In the lapels of their jackets they wear a badge: less than a thumbnail's width in diameter, as small as the Légion d'Honneur and worn with equal pride, it was designed by two Americans in Dacca, Bangladesh.

The association is the "Order of the Bifurcated Needle." The inventor of the original needle, Dr. Ben Rubin, director of research at the Wyeth Laboratories in the United States, received the John Scott Award for it in 1981, a distinction given every year since the late 1700s for an eminent invention, but he describes this tool as "possibly one of the least consequential things I've ever done." Yet the needle was one of the most important tools in human history, for it underpinned the most magnificent achievement in the history of medicine: the global eradication of smallpox. Between its two prongs it held a minute drop of vaccine and, when quickly tapped some fifteen times on a person's arm, delivered a small dose of live virus under the skin. One day, using a pair of pliers the two Americans bent the prongs into a zero and the logo and badge came to symbolize the motto for the entire campaign: *Smallpox Zero.*

Small is not always beautiful. Two varieties of smallpox exist, *Variola minor* and *Variola major,* and both are caused by a minute virus whose diameter is a mere 200 thousandths of an inch. The diameter of the earth is 507 million inches. Yet the effects of the one on the history of the other is of a magnitude just as great as the ratio of their different sizes. As smallpox raged in epidemics and pandemics, its ravages determined the course of human history and by the eighteenth century few places or people had escaped. It killed Chinese emperors, African tribal kings, European monarchs, Arab potentates, and millions of unknown people. By decimating the native populations, smallpox enabled the Spanish to conquer Mexico, and white settlers the Native Americans, they called the "Indians." But by decimating their own army it also prevented those very same settlers from capturing Canada. In the eighteenth century smallpox caused one-third of all blindness in Europe; in the nineteenth, 400,000 Europeans were dying from it every year. By the midtwentieth century, ten to fifteen million people in thirty-three countries were succumbing, with two million dying each year.

After a person has been first infected with smallpox, the virus incubates for up to fourteen days, then fever, headaches, and vomiting begin. Three days later a characteristic rash erupts and then scabs form, which, when they fall off, leave unpigmented, pockmarked areas of skin. There is no treatment: in the virulent form, 20 percent of all victims died and 1 percent of the survivors were left blind. Death rates were always highest in young children; the infection gathered in pustules, the children bled, and the pain was so severe that they could not move.

The eradication of smallpox was a triumph that chalked up several firsts, yet it was still "a damned close-run thing." All the necessary elements for success were available – a vaccine, a methodology, a commitment, and a campaign – but one element was, of course, an absolute prerequisite. Edward Jenner, a doctor practicing in southwest England in the eighteenth century, first tried vaccination on May 14, 1796. By inoculating people with harmless cowpox, he gave them immunity to smallpox, but alone that proved little. Jenner's genius lay in demonstrating their acquired immunity in an experiment that today would never be permitted. He inoculated these same people with active smallpox virus and showed that they were now protected.

Centuries before, it had been observed that those who survived smallpox never caught it again and a protective practice, *variolation,* emerged which never entirely died out. Variolators ranged through the countryside, carrying scabs and pus to scratch into the skin: in Turkey young children were regularly assembled for variolation; in India, Brahmin priests traveled around offering prayers to the goddess of smallpox and variolation to the people. But, one may ask, since live smallpox virus was in the pus, how could variolation protect? It appears that when smallpox infection comes by inoculation through the skin, the fatality rate is only one-tenth of that which occurs when the virus is passed naturally. We still don't know why and so, in places like Ethiopia, where the virus strain was mild, variolation caused few problems. But in Afghanistan, where the strain was the virulent *Variola major,* swathes of epidemics followed the variolators and soon the practice was forbidden with punishments meted out to those who tried it.

Once vaccination existed, however, eradication of the disease was theoretically possible. Indeed, in 1806, the president of the United States, Thomas Jefferson, wrote to Dr. Edward Jenner: "Future nations will know by history only that the loathsome smallpox has existed and by you has been exterpated." Today, all children under eight years of age know smallpox by "history only," but it took far longer than Thomas Jefferson ever imagined to get rid of this disease.

It shouldn't have taken so long, for many factors worked in favor of eradication of the virus. For a start the smallpox virus is "an honourable gentleman among infectious agents," one comparatively simple to eradicate for the symptoms were obvious, the disease easily identified without laboratory tests, the rash characteristic, and patients only infectious for four days before it appeared. Moreover almost permanent immunity followed an infection or vaccination. Finally, the virus could not survive for long outside a human being and this was to be its Achilles' heel. Prevent the virus being passed from person to person and the disease would die out. Since infection spread slowly, with an incubation period of up to two weeks, there was plenty of time for the crucial intervention.

The epidemiology also helped. The only people at risk from smallpox were those who had both neither had smallpox nor a successful vaccination, *and* who came into actual contact with an infected person. Only a fraction of a susceptible population would fulfill these conditions. This was why, once vaccination was routine, outbreaks in the developed countries were easily controlled. It was simply a matter of finding the cases, then quickly tracing and vaccinating their contacts.

The nature of the vaccine, too, was crucial: it was safe and highly effective and gave superb protection. Though ideally it should be refrigerated, it can survive for one month if kept cool and since it can be freeze-dried like a yogurt culture, transport is no problem. Once shaken up in sterile water or saline solution, it is ready. The device to deliver it was equally effective: a simple scratching "fork" was displaced by a rapid-fire jet-gun, which in turn gave way to the bifurcated needle that delivered just one drop and needed neither repair nor maintenance. But the technology for global eradication was at hand long before the commitment, the cash, and the international cooperation.

It was not until after the Second World War that attempts began to bring all these elements together. Though vaccination was widespread, smallpox was still endemic in many countries. National vaccination programs were mounted virtually everywhere, even in those countries where the disease was not endemic, simply to prevent major outbreaks should the disease be reintroduced, and mandatory vaccination certificates were generally required for all travelers. The administrative fuss and bother were a great nuisance and the costs were high. For example, in 1969 it was estimated that to vaccinate or revaccinate the population of the United States, and provide treatment for those, who, as a result, had complications, cost $150 million a year – and still the disease continued to flourish.

Then, in 1958, at the World Health Organization Assembly, the USSR delegate proposed that smallpox eradication be undertaken as a formal commitment of WHO. One year later the organization agreed and many mass vaccination programs were started. By the middle of the decade, the project had run aground however. Poor countries just could not undertake campaigns; others found their efforts thwarted as war and the movements of refugees carried smallpox from place to place; sufficient vaccine did not exist, nor was it always effective. As their programs faltered, the endemic countries became disheartened and even in those that claimed successful mass vaccination, smallpox was flaring again. Then malaria eradication programs, which had been widespread since the war, began to stall too and this led to widespread skepticism about eradicating anything.

The crunch came in the mid-1960s when forty-four countries were reporting smallpox, and it was endemic in thirty-three. In one year alone, though only 131,000 cases were officially reported, some ten to fifteen million actually occurred. So now the WHO Assembly decided that global eradication should either be quietly forgotten or properly attempted and in 1966 the delegates asked for additional money – $2.5 million – a mere 5 percent of that year's WHO budget and, over the protests of the director general, got it. They called for a "ten-year campaign" that unconsciously mirrored Kennedy's program to land a man on the moon within a decade. Indeed, some delegates did comment, "If you can land a man on the moon in the ten years, why can't we eradicate smallpox in the same time?" So WHO set about finding someone to direct the campaign. The man chosen was an American, Dr. Donald A. Henderson, widely and affectionately known as D. A. This was a job, he now says, that he absolutely did *not* want.

One day, so we are promised, Dr. Henderson, now dean of the School of Public Health at Johns Hopkins University, Baltimore, Maryland, will tell his own story of the years that ensued. It will be worth waiting for, though he admits it might be impossible to reveal all. Brought in from the outside and pitched straight into the battle, he remained the campaign's general to the very end. His style, personality, and formidable strengths were absolutely crucial to its success.

When Henderson's posting came, he was busy setting up a smallpox eradication and measles control program in West Africa. As he commuted between Europe, Africa, and the United States – obtaining support, developing operational plans, and explaining their details to the West African countries, signing agreements, organizing materials, recruiting people – he was acquiring skills that later would stand him in good stead: maneuvering tactfully through bureaucratic jungles, treading gingerly through political minefields. All was in place when suddenly he was called in by the U.S. Surgeon-General and told to drop everything and fly to Geneva to direct global smallpox eradication. Henderson was aghast. He felt a responsibility to the people already recruited. To leave them so soon seemed wrong. The West African program was problem enough without having the whole world placed in his hands, and he was already thoroughly disturbed by the bureaucratic struggles at WHO. Many people questioned whether that organization could ever execute *anything*.

Thus, when the Surgeon-General dropped his bombshell, Henderson protested: "The Public Health Service is not run like the army. There's always been discussion, then mutual agreement."

"You are ordered to go in this case."

"Suppose I refuse?"

"Well, you could always resign."

"Great heavens, are you serious?"

"Yes, we are," came the implacable reply.

A compromise was reached. If in the first eighteen months, Henderson decided his position was impossible, he would send a cable with the single word "NOW" and they would extricate him. So certain was he that his time overseas would be measured in months that his family took only half of their household goods to Geneva. They stayed eleven years.

Although the flesh may not have been willing, the spirit was not entirely unwilling. Indeed many colleagues now say that Henderson really wanted the job all along and for one simple reason: he actually believed smallpox eradication *was* possible. Transmission had already been interrupted in a number of countries and in others the disease had been eradicated. A good vaccine existed, so if the resources were available, why could it not be done? Publicly, Henderson always expressed confidence, but privately he was uneasy about motivation and commitment. Moreover, he took seriously the skepticism about smallpox eradication expressed by rational scientists whose opinions he respected. The biologist, Dr. René Dubos, for example, had written that even if there were no "theoretical flaws" and "technical difficulties" in such programs, "earthly factors would certainly bring them soon to a gentle and silent death. Certain unpleasant, but universal human traits will put impassable stumbling blocks on the road to eradication."

So Henderson was not at all surprised when, like a swarm of angry bees, a multitude of problems immediately descended on his head and remained there for the next eleven years. His daily skirmishes ran the gamut: the frustrating attitudes common to any bureaucracy but often exaggerated to the highest absurdity in international agencies. He smoothed the ruffled feathers and territorial conflicts that had been caused by appointment of an American as director of the campaign. Conflicts arose over his making appointments on the basis of professional skills rather than on equal representation of nationalities. Hauteur was provoked when he objected to unsatisfactory staff being dumped on his program. D. A. battled to overcome the reluctance of the WHO regional directors to appoint special smallpox advisers in their areas; four did so promptly, but the other two gave the job to busy individuals who had many other responsibilities besides. He assuaged the scandalized pain provoked by his prompt setting of such precedents as a research budget under his control and a regular means of communicating with his people. And if these were not enough, there were problems that had never been expected.

The vaccine caused a big headache, for only a small proportion already in use met any standards at all, whether of cleanliness or immunological potency. Henderson was adamant: he didn't care where it came from, all vaccine had to be independently monitored. Never before had anyone had the temerity to challenge the quality standards of other countries, but finally the WHO Assembly agreed: only vaccines tested by independent monitoring laboratories in Canada or the Netherlands would be used. This decision hurt national pride, but many countries soon changed their production methods.

The next problem was to mobilize at least 250 million doses every year. With a budget of just $2 million, Henderson couldn't afford these even at one cent a dose. The Soviets offered large quantities for use in India, and another 25 million doses to be sent wherever he wanted; the Americans gave vaccine for the whole West Africa program. But most endemic countries would eventually produce their own, using foreign consultants to help develop the commercial methods and guarantee quality.

Having faced WHO, Henderson turned outward to persuade, cajole, seduce, promise, or appeal to those countries with epidemic smallpox to undertake eradication programs. Formal agreements had to be signed with every single one; some were achieved easily, some not. The first moment of "near absolute catastrophe," he says, occurred in Nigeria where he planned a regional headquarters. More than half of the people he had recruited would be assigned to Western and Central Africa, for the size of the population demanded this. But as the equipment was actually being loaded, Nigeria was slowly drifting into civil war. Desperate approaches were made to the country's president through every diplomatic channel, and all met a flat refusal. Finally Henderson sent Dr. George Lythcott, who would be his regional director for West Africa and ultimately head of the Health Services Administrative Agency in Washington, "a diplomat in Accra at that time, and a very imaginative guy," he says. His instructions were to go out there and "get it, somehow or other." Every night for a week or so, Lythcott telephoned in the small hours, but there was no progress. Ten days had gone by before finally he called and said, "Signed. I'm on my way back."

"What happened?" asked Henderson and got the reply: "I can't tell you now and I'm not sure I ever will tell you." But one day he did. He cultivated Nigerian society extensively and, quite by chance, wound up at a party one Saturday night where he was introduced to the girlfriend of a high government official. Paramours have often played vital and honorable roles in history, and this was one such occasion. She heard the story on Saturday and the agreement was signed on Monday.

Although these particular circumstances were never again repeated, there were many such cliff-hangers, and the strategies necessary to resolve them were different in each country. Finally, all agreements were signed. Later gossip was inaccurate: no bribes or payments were ever offered. They would not have been helpful and, in any case, the program didn't have any spare cash!

Recruiting the epidemiologists was the least of Henderson's problems. He wanted the best people and made certain that he got them. Some, like the American Bill Foege, he had known from earlier days in

Atlanta. Others, like the Englishman Nick Ward, he recruited wherever he found them. Ward, a tall, thin man with a sensitive vulnerability hidden deep under a tough competence, had gone to a remote swamp in northern Botswana to see "the biggest crocodiles" in Africa, and to keep himself occupied, had taken a local team to do smallpox vaccination as well. When Henderson turned up, everybody had already been vaccinated, not only in the local village but in all the surrounding ones, too. Henderson, most impressed, found out who was responsible, called him and said, "Why don't you come and work for me?" So Nick Ward ended up in the program, as did Claudio do Amaral, a Brazilian; Daniel Tarantola and Nicole Grasset, French; Ali Naggar Mourad, Egyptian; Khim Mu Aye, Burmese; Ludmilla Tchicherchukzna, Russian; Dr. Kamarul Huda and Abu Yusuf, Bangladeshis – just a few of the seven hundred or so men and women who were finally recruited. Their quality was superb and so too was their commitment, but then, so too was the leadership.

For eleven years, Henderson's concerns would cover the spectrum of human experience, from vision to venality. He describes his life as weekly episodes of the "Perils of Pauline" and he could never guess what problem would surface at any time. One of his staff, Dr. do Amaral, was kidnapped in Ethiopia at a time of the border war. He had already been badly injured, having been neatly, but luckily not fatally, scalped by a helicopter blade. Henderson recalls,

"WHO and the Ethiopian government had agreed that no ransoms would ever be paid – not that we had any money. God knows, we hardly had enough for supplies. But access to the rebel groups is generally quite easy in these places. There will be local people who have brothers or friends or uncles, who know someone in the market who knows someone else, whose uncle's cousin belongs to one of the rebel groups. So the message filtered down: there isn't a cent for anything, so please send the guy home."

Eventually the kidnappers agreed, but not before do Amaral had lined them all up and had tapped every one of them fifteen times with his bifurcated needle. Only then did he allow them to let him go!

Money was a persistent worry. People later carped that there was no way the campaign could have failed since Henderson bulldozed his way through every problem, which he sometimes did, and had unlimited resources, which he did not. The vaccine was either purchased from drug companies and then donated, or produced in the endemic countries. Wyeth Laboratories waived all patent rights on the bifurcated needles and supplied them below cost. But the program director had "a devil of a time" getting financial support from any government in the developed countries, with three exceptions: the United States, Sweden, and the Soviet Union. Although twenty-six other countries did make small contributions in cash or kind, there was no support at all from the remainder. "I went hat in hand everywhere," Henderson says, "begging for money, and getting it by flukey circumstances rather than any rational decision-making process."

Commitment was equally worrying, Henderson now says:

There's another myth that those countries where smallpox was endemic were *eager* to undertake smallpox eradication. Not true. Even though they had all gone to the World Health Assembly and had voted the program the highest priority, most, when approached, said, "So what?" The African and most Asian countries just weren't interested. It was a real pain and we were in a very tight situation. I can name point after point where the program hung by a thread, where, if it had not been for this person, or for that situation, or for this rescue, we would have failed. A change of government at the wrong point, a civil war erupting when we least expected it and we were down the tube. We got rid of smallpox in Uganda, then Idi Amin created havoc. Things quieted down just long enough for us to go in and make sure smallpox was really gone, and then all hell broke loose again. We did it when we could, and if we hadn't done it then, I doubt we would have done it at all.

Though Donald A. Henderson and his colleagues would finally surmount every obstacle, solve every problem, there was one country where the outcome persistently hung by a thread. Had this battle been lost, the entire global effort would have foundered. Yet, paradoxically, in August 1970, at the peak of the campaign's success, this country was entirely free of smallpox.

The summer of 1970 marked an important moment in the campaign to eradicate smallpox, because it was the time when the focus shifted from Africa, where smallpox transmission had been almost totally severed, to Asia. The number of *reported* cases in Asia was small, but the hiding of smallpox was rife, and between twenty and two hundred times more cases were actually occurring than the number officially proclaimed. D. A. and his Geneva staff knew that they didn't have to worry about one country at least – East Pakistan – for there really *was* no smallpox. A good health infrastructure existed, staffed by skilled and devoted workers, and vaccination programs had been in operation for nine years. Then between 1968 and 1971, a brilliant and imaginative final campaign, intensively conducted by these workers and led by two WHO officials, Dr. Isao Arita, Japanese, and Dr. Karl Markvart, Czechoslovakian, finished off the job.

For twenty-three years since 1947, when the British finally left India, East Pakistan remained physically separated from its other half, West Pakistan. Having 1,500 miles of foreign territory between its two capital cities, Dacca and Rawalpindi, caused endless strains, and eventually the political and civil tensions became intolerable. Civil war broke out and on December 16, 1971, East Pakistan was "liberated," becoming Bangladesh.

The country is formed by the land between three huge rivers — the Ganges, Meghna, and Brahmaputra — that join in a massive deltaic plain. Half of Bangladesh consists of water; the rest is flat land formed from the silt and topsoil carried down each year as the waters of the Himalayas surge across the land. Catastrophic flooding is a regular feature of life, and only the southeastern region escapes, where a few steeply sloping hills rise to 3,000 feet. So Bangladesh is a land of vast horizons and great skies whose canopy sweeps right down to eye level. The horizon is quickly dwarfed by storm clouds towering higher and higher into the sky. Most areas receive two hundred inches of rain each year; even those considered dry get fifty inches, and it all pours down in a single spell of three months. When the monsoon breaks in mid-June, existence becomes strings, sheets, curtains of torrential rain that can beat down nonstop for six days at a time and with such force that the drops bounce to waist level. A stretch of twenty-five miles that can be walked in April will be under eight feet of water in June. So the difference between normality and catastrophe is only a few feet.

In the deltaic plain, where rice and jute are farmed, the land is one of familiar reflections: oxen ploughing the paddies; peasants bowing to their mirrored images as, ankle deep in water, they transplant rice seedlings; children darting down to scoop for little fish directly from the mud. If the rivers are the lifeblood of the country — a vast, autonomous infrastructure supporting millions through transport, commerce, or fishing — its blood corpuscles are the boats, either small ferries, country boats, or stately galleons that, carrying one massive sail, glide effortlessly downstream drifting with the current.

In the cities, the bicycle rickshaws are to the streets what the boats are to the streams. Straining arms, pounding hearts, and aching muscles provide the force that drives Bangladesh, whether applied to a load of hay dragged down a country lane or to people pulled across a city street, or to the boats now loaded and hauled back upstream foot by foot.

As a consequence it is difficult to find a fat person in Bangladesh and if you do, he or she will either be a foreigner, a bureaucrat, or a merchant.

Life is precarious, people everywhere poor, but though Bangladesh is small, only two-thirds the size of Florida, in 1971 it supported 75 million people. By 1984 there were 92 million. By train you can travel from one end of the country to the other in just one day. Some people don't even buy a ticket; along with hundreds of others, they cling to the sides of the carriages or climb on the roof (or did so before it was forbidden). Others mount bullock carts, or grasp buses, just another unit added to a dynamic, fragile, mobile, human pyramid.

That smallpox had suddenly reappeared in Bangladesh was realized not on the spot, but in the United States. When Pakistan's civil war began, ten million people fled to India and were housed in refugee camps. A staff member of the Center for Disease Control in Atlanta, watching a television news film, spotted smallpox on the faces of the refugees. CDC telexed Donald Henderson in Geneva, who immediately telexed his people in Delhi, who in turn telexed Calcutta and teams rushed to the camp. But they were too late; before containment could begin, the war ended and the local administrators just piled the refugees onto the transports and shipped them back to Bangladesh, even though many had active smallpox. Rapidly the people fanned out into the southwest corner of the country. Khulna was the first town to be overwhelmed, then Dacca, and soon there wasn't a single chain of infection but *thousands*. By January 1972, Dr. Nilton Arnt, a Brazilian physician monitoring Bangladesh, realized matters were getting out of control. He needed help urgently and Dr. Nick Ward was posted to him. They faced chaos. Everything, from transport to supplies, had broken down; all administrative structures were disrupted and the health services all but wrecked. There were still a few brilliant planners and bureaucrats in Dacca, ready to formulate strategy, and there were still thousands of health workers in the field ready to execute it. But there was no effective communication between the two groups, and since there was total administrative collapse at the local level, only foreigners were able to forge the necessary links.

This situation was immediately reflected in an appalling, catastrophic surge of smallpox. Containment proved fruitless, for now as before, there was little incentive for the poor to report the disease. Reporting might be suppressed either through fatalism (people believed smallpox was the regular result of the spring visit from the goddess of smallpox) or through personal pride. A few local civil surgeons fostered the hiding of cases, fearing these would reflect on their efficiency. So as administration and control disappeared, the disease gained a stranglehold on the country, and the magnificent achievement of the past nine years melted away in a few short weeks.

During that year and into 1973, Dr. Ward was responsible for the campaign in Bangladesh. To understand the strategy that now developed and which over the next four years became beautifully refined, it is important to understand two closely linked factors. Both were crucial. The first relates to the seasons. Smallpox always peaked in January and February, when the disease spread like wildfire. Then the numbers fell away and just why this happened, no one knew then or knows now. But as new cases became fewer, the trick would be to find them all, isolate the patients, and vaccinate their contacts. With this falling curve of numbers, the chain of human-to-human infection could be snapped.

The second crucial factor is the cities. Although less than 5 percent of Bangladeshis live in urban areas, the cities influence the spread of the disease out of all proportion to their size. This is because in times of catastrophe and stress, people pour into the cities, particularly into Dacca, seeking food, shelter, and work, and when the crisis is over, they all pour out again. Even permanent city dwellers, when ill, return to the comfort and reassurance of their families in the countryside. So, seething with humanity, Dacca is a centrifuge ceaselessly spinning its population, with some people being drawn into the center while others are shot out to the circumference. The vast majority of those flocking in are the poorest of all, who are forced to live in the densely crowded slums, the *bastis*.

These two factors, springtime and the cities, are closely linked by a third, the weather. If Nature is kind just enough rain occurs for a bountiful harvest but not enough for a catastrophic flood. So people stay put. But Bangladesh is frequently not so blessed. Famine and flood were everyone's enemies in the war against smallpox, causing poor people to migrate, the urban centrifuge to spin faster and faster, and the spiral of infection to intensify.

In 1971 and early 1972, the ending of the civil war played the same role as catastrophic floods. Within days the refugees had moved from the southwest corner of the country to Dacca and the spiral was started. The special character of Dacca now exacerbated the problem. The city is a maze of alleyways, markets, streets, and bazaars that spreads over some thirty square miles, slashed by one railway line, two rivers, and some half-dozen highways. Traffic is hopelessly undisciplined: rickshaws weave recklessly in and out of bus lanes; buses, overloaded and decrepit, smash their way through intersections; trucks apparently held by rope and willpower cross all double lines, willing and ready to do battle with the oncoming traffic; cars honking their horns wildly, crawl down the old streets in any direction according to the driver's whim, judgment, or illusions of virility; pedestrians, burdened by worry, children, and commercial loads, scurry in and out as fatalistically and as determinedly as any other moving entity; and in vain do the traffic cops blow their whistles and wave their arms.

Dacca is a dangerous place, but not because you might get mugged. No matter how you travel, the indiscriminately moving mass that pushes and shoves and crashes can knock you down, run you over, and turn you into just one more statistic. There are so many moving people in any street that you can never see where you are going and unless you know your destination, it will be a miracle if you ever arrive. Yet now Nick Ward deliberately set out to study Dacca and came to know it better than anyone ever before and perhaps since.

Unlike most cities, Dacca never flaunts its wealth; it is poverty that is abundant and obvious, and this was another crucial factor in small-pox control. Those at the bottom of the heap, housed under strips of cloth that pass for roofs, which are somehow attached to corrugated tin sections that pass for walls, live as best they can. They scavenge, and the garbage of those higher up the human chain provide the sustenance for those farther down. Yet though most of the returning refugees who, in 1972, now piled into Dacca, lived in the shanties strung out along the railway line, or in the congested bastis, at least one million found no permanent resting place at all. Two hundred thousand people actually moved in and out of the city *each* day, and since it was spring, the period of highest smallpox transmission, there was soon a massive epidemic. Each day 800 of these transients caught smallpox, 2,500 died, and that meant there were probably 15,000 cases in all during this first period. There was no way that the health workers could control such an epidemic: trying to find the patients, isolate them, and selectively vaccinate their contacts was hopeless. Certainly they posted guards at burial grounds, ferry terminals, railway stations, hospitals, health clinics, "shooting" everyone with the jet guns of vaccine, and tried to trace all cases back to their sources – but the task was impossible. Nick Ward felt that they had no alternative but to try and vaccinate en masse, on a house-to-house basis, in the slums and along the railway line. By the time this first epidemic subsided, three million people had been vaccinated in Dacca.

Throughout the next four years, Dacca would be the nightmare the health workers could not dispel, the reality they could not grasp. They would come to know the rural areas and the movements of people between villages well enough to control most outbreaks. But in those terrible early months of 1972, Ward rightly saw his priority to get the cities free and worry about the countryside later.

Another person now joined them. That in January 1972, Dr. Stan Foster from the Center for Disease Control, Atlanta, was recruited was pure luck and, Ward says, one of the best things that could have happened. He and Nilton Arnt were off to Delhi for one of the meetings that Donald Henderson regularly called. Foster was visiting Bangladesh on a nutrition survey and Ward asked him to keep an eye on smallpox while they were away. Being a very active man as well as an extremely competent epidemiologist, Foster began surveying Dacca and soon discovered a massive outbreak. Now they had two tasks: to locate the focal points where the disease was erupting and to reconstitute the program that had successfully controlled the disease in the years before the nation's independence. Many more Bangladeshis and foreigners were rapidly recruited.

Mobile surveillance teams formed the core of the new campaign. There were six in that first year, 1972 – 1973, but by 1975 there would be fifty. At first supervised by foreigners, the teams were eventually totally composed of and led by Bangladeshis. These people did the bulk of the work, whether surveillance and vaccinating, or statistics and treatment, or logistics and liaison. The heart of their activity remained throughout, however, the finding of cases, the tracing of contacts, and vaccination. Their numbers constantly expanded; all had a secondary school education. At the start there were 175 in Dacca, but within four years 300 were working in the city alone. There would finally be 12,000 on the payroll across the country and if those who manned the necessary supporting infrastructure were also included, the number would be 25,000.

The work was arduous and the time demanded so great that soon a joke began circulating in Dacca: "The best form of birth control is to join the smallpox program." But those working in the city could at least go home at night. It was a quite different matter for those posted to the countryside, where most of the foreigners ended up.

From a distance the small villages of Bangladesh stand out on slight eminences like sand castles on rounded heaps, with the village boundaries clearly defined, whether by canals feeding a rice paddy, or streams crossed by bridges formed from rods of suspended bamboo. Each village has a schoolhouse and a central pond where people wash themselves, their clothes, and their animals. The well-defined mud tracks that serve as streets churn sticky in the rainy season. Dotted through the compound along their lengths are tea shops and booths, where people sell miscellaneous metal goods, or herbal remedies, or an assortment of canned foods. In their own way these villages are quite as crowded as Dacca, and though the human numbers were far more manageable, the conditions in which the foreigners lived were far more primitive, sometimes appalling.

In the country motorbikes and feet carried the health workers from rumor to confirmation, from report to patient. The rice paddies, threshing floors, schools, mosques, bus stops, the paths along the railway lines, were their beats. They would start very early every morning, often cold, for damp fog blankets the delta in the winter and spring, and always tired. They would have slept on the thin bedrolls carried strapped to their bikes, lying on the floors, benches, or tables of the government *dak* bungalows, if there were any, in ordinary huts if not. They were kept moving for twenty-five days at a stretch and then they had five days off. A normal working day involved following up all reports, and contacting the local leaders – the *mullahs,* politicians, healers, teachers – all of whom were influential and a good source of further information. Wherever they found themselves, the objective was the same: to uncover all the active cases, isolate them until the infectious period was past, and vaccinate all contacts.

This procedure was strikingly different from that of earlier smallpox programs, when mass vaccination had been the official strategy and success measured by the total numbers vaccinated. But under Donald Henderson's rule, the number of *new* cases occurring now became the index of progress, or failure. The headquarters staff at WHO in Geneva – composed of D. A. Henderson, Isao Arita, and Jock Copland, who stayed together for the entire campaign, focused on improved reporting as the key for their strategy. They anticipated that it would take at least three years before a system of surveillance and containment would be developed efficient enough to break the chain of transmission and they expected that they would still have to vaccinate at least 80 percent of any given population.

This is better than 100 percent, but in Bangladesh, it represented a massive 63 million people. Then the program had a lucky break. In a combination of chance and brilliance, Bill Foege discovered that it was not necessary to vaccinate even 80 percent. He was directing the campaign in Eastern Nigeria, where there was an extensive missionary network with radios that linked the mission stations. Using these airways, Foege could learn about smallpox cases very quickly and soon had developed a sophisticated reporting system. Then one month, his supplies were delayed and he had urgently to reassess his priorities. He decided to concentrate solely on the containment of *known* outbreaks and in a blanket operation searched them out and vaccinated everyone in one small area around each case. By the time his supplies finally arrived six months later, he could find no more smallpox, yet *less than 50 percent* of his population had been vaccinated.

Although the number that needed to be vaccinated in order to break transmission varied from country to country, it turned out to be far less than anyone ever guessed. In remote, sparsely populated regions of Africa, transmission could be stopped with a much lower coverage than in regions of tightly packed, mobile individuals. Thus the task facing the teams in Bangladesh was of a different order of magnitude from the task in, say, Ethiopia. Nevertheless, Bill Foege's contribution was the single most significant breakthrough in the whole campaign. Not only was the new procedure highly effective, it also reduced labor, supplies, and cost.

Thus, armed with an expanded staff and a new method, the countrywide campaign in Bangladesh sprang into gear again in mid-1972. The teams first relied on reporting techniques devised by a health worker in Indonesia. All the successful techniques, in fact, would be suggested by local people. They would hold up a photograph of a baby covered with smallpox and ask: "Do you know anyone who looks like this?" If the answer was yes, they went to the suspected patient as quickly as they could, taking their informant along too. Says Stan Foster,

We soon learned that within the catchment area of a market, which could be twenty-five square miles, about 80 percent of the smallpox cases would be found. So our first attempts were inquiries in places where people collected, like markets or ferry docks or railroad stations. Markets took place about once every five days and the team would try to hit all the major markets within one area. Only males came and they soon found that young boys eight to thirteen were the best reporters, less reluctant to "rat" on their neighbors than older people, and you could tell more by the expression on a child's face than from his words. There was that instant glimmer of recognition which meant "I have seen this."

Rapidly their campaign gathered momentum. Then suddenly Khulna, the second largest city in Bangladesh once again became swamped with smallpox, with cases originating in its slums being passed out to the villages. On the borders with India, too, the disease was still spreading like wildfire. Though the medical officers and health workers were excellent, they had far too much to do, being responsible for malaria, nutrition, and intestinal disease as well as smallpox; therefore only a minute percentage of cases was being reported. One group in the country, still loyal to Pakistan, the Biharis, were awaiting repatriation (they still are), seeking food and work, the men moved to the city and caught smallpox. As a minority under suspicion and frightened of the authorities, the Biharis hid their disease and so smallpox quickly raged through their camps too. Nick Ward recalls:

One camp in Muhammedpur contained 10,000 people and we found two cases of smallpox. I decided to vaccinate the whole camp and in two days we did just that. Ten days later, on the mandatory follow-up visit, I found an unvaccinated girl who had just given birth to stillborn twins: all three had smallpox. I blew my top. "Why wasn't this girl vaccinated?" "Oh, she was pregnant," I was told. "We thought it wouldn't be nice to vaccinate her." And of course, pregnancy and smallpox don't go too well together, so she died.

In another camp of 120,000 Biharis, there were five cases. We found them, vaccinated their contacts, and put them in our little isolation hospital. Returning a couple of days later we found the hospital empty. They had run away in the middle of the night because they did not want to be separated from their families. Single acts like these put you back two or more weeks. From those five people *alone* the next generation of cases totaled 198 people. This time we called in both the Red Cross and all the WHO people and again we vaccinated 120,000 people in one weekend.

But not everyone wished to be vaccinated, refusing because of fear, religious belief, apathy, or fatalism. No one could possibly banish smallpox and, in any case, why did these foreigners ignore the sick and do something only to the healthy; why indeed were they concentrating just on the spring disease, when there were many more important problems around, hunger for a start?

For those whose job it was to eradicate smallpox, the situation was acutely distressing. On every side people were dying, and the health-workers' very real sensitivities to the objections of those who refused vaccination conflicted with the certain knowledge that if they didn't vaccinate, smallpox would never disappear. An American doctor, Larry Brilliant, has written poignantly about these conflicts. When the Asian campaign began, he was in an ashram in the Himalayan foothills seeking spiritual guidance from an aged ascetic guru. After one year there he was mightily surprised to receive not only the compassionate spirituality he had expected, but one firm, practical injunction: he and his wife were to go and work in the villages giving vaccinations, for smallpox would be eradicated in India. Thus he found himself one night watching as an Indian government team broke into an adobe hut in a village where vaccination was being fiercely resisted, and a man and his entire family were forcibly vaccinated against the verbal and physical protests of Mohan Singh, the leader of the local

Ho tribe. When, panting and exhausted, each group finally faced each other, Mohan Singh broke the tension by quietly walking to his vegetable plot, picking the only cucumber on the vine and, in a gesture of traditional hospitality, handing it to the Indian doctor, whom his wife had just bitten. Then lit by the first red rays of the morning sun, Mohan Singh said:

Only God can decide who gets sickness and who does not. It is my duty to resist your interference with his will. We must resist your needles. We have done our duty; you say you act in accordance with your duty. It is over. God will decide. Now I find you are guests in my house. It is my duty to feed guests. I have little to offer at this time except this cucumber.

Emotionally numb, Brilliant momentarily wondered whose side he was on and it was his Muslim paramedical assistant, Zafar Hussain, who, humbly bowing before Mohan Singh, spoke for new attitudes and changes in belief:

You live by God's will. I, too, have surrendered to God's will. These vaccinators are of your tribe. They also share your faith. But what is God's will? Is it God's will that you go hungry or that you plant rice and eat? Is it God's will that you go naked or that you make cloth and cover yourself? Look around you at your children. How many are absent today, dead from smallpox? That one over there is blind forever. Smallpox can be stopped with this vaccine. Must we all produce four children so that two will survive smallpox? I think it is God's will that our people don't suffer any more . . . that we take vaccination. It is my *dharma* to protect your children from smallpox.

Taking hold of Brilliant's arm, Zafar Hussain vaccinated him, for about the hundredth time, and then beckoned an elderly man on the fringe of the crowd and pleaded gently: "We are not the enemy. Please take vaccination." The man stepped forward and, in the dawn, five hundred villagers were immunized.

Similar scenes were to occur over and over, but to begin with the foreigners did not have the gentle subtlety of Zafar Hussain. Nick Ward explains what impelled their actions and attitudes.

In the early stages, for perhaps two or three years, the urgency made us much more physical, much more anxious to push on, in spite of – very often in direct contravention of – what the people wanted us to do. There were, of course, problems on both sides. For a start, in the Islamic faith, it is very difficult for anybody in the house except the man to take decisions. If he'd gone away you would not be allowed to enter the house, let alone see the cases and vaccinate mothers and children. You could only do this if the man was there to give permission. If he wasn't, you could do one of two things: either insist and try to get the neighbors to help you, or go away and come back in a week's time. The first wasn't always very easy, for people didn't want to cause trouble, especially if they were from a minority group. They also thought that the patient would be taken away to the hospital and all sorts of people would be trampling around, and when their man returned, he would be very angry indeed. So as well as simply running out of the back door and disappearing into the bush, they hid people. If you didn't insist on going into the house *and* looking in every room *and* under the beds *and* in the privies, you were certainly going to miss cases. When you did search the house, people would run off to the bottom of the garden, where the privy was (a little house on stilts). The door would be locked and the neighbors would say, "There is somebody on the toilet. Don't bother there." But if you got on your hands and knees and looked up through the hole from beneath, you could see eight pairs of legs, all squashed inside. So of course you had to go in and vaccinate everybody in those cramped, crowded surroundings.

We had this screaming problem, you see. *People were dying*. Did we just sit back and do it the gentle way we would have liked, but knew wouldn't work, or did we just bulldoze? We got to the situation in Dacca where we knew we just had to immunize *everybody*, because of the crowds always coming in and going out. You literally had to do 200,000 people a day *just to stand still*.

Containment in such a place was terribly difficult though. The city people were magnificent, giving us all the support we needed, and although I always speak as if *we* were doing it, of course it was the Bangladesh and the Dacca municipal people who were actually doing it. In the mornings they would vaccinate all the people they could in a given area, but still 40 percent of the people would not be found. The children had run away; the women had hidden.

In the end [Ward continued, ruefully], I did something I'm not particularly proud of, but it was a fact of life at the time. We organized a band of vigilantes, about forty-four white, foreign infidels who were not likely to be excessively worried about the finer points of Muslim belief – wives of our own people, schoolteachers, visitors, and sometimes their children – all volunteers. We would transport them around the city in the afternoons. They were phenomenally good. It was their job to get the usual 60 percent coverage as high as they could and very often they got it up to 100 percent. Stan Foster's eldest son, Willie, used to go out looking for cases when he was home on holiday. He and his father would vaccinate the slums together and far from resenting this, the Bengalis loved Willie.

We nearly lost some of our people, though. Somebody *was* killed with an arrow in India, and another had his head slit open with a cleaver. One person turned up who had heard George Harrison's song, "Bangladesh" and decided that he ought to come to help this new nation. He was vaccinating with Nilton Arnt along the disused railway line in the old city – a mass of bamboo and polythene shacks, chock full of people. One old woman was furious, but he had just moved on from her to the next person when Arnt walked into the shed, dived, and pulled her arm away, as she raised her axe to bring it down on top of the foreigner's head.

But since the local people, as good Muslims, didn't feel they could go barging into another man's house they were virtually never assaulted, because they were always very polite and respectful. They were doing what was the right thing, what now we with hindsight would do.

The most remarkable fact of these two, punishing years, 1972-1973, was their constant, euphoric and totally misplaced optimism. For as they realize now, by the end of 1972, they actually knew only 10 percent of all existing cases. Their optimism might have been misplaced but it was not unjustified. As Nick Ward says:

You could see the results – smallpox disappearing in the areas where you were working. In 1973 we split up the country. Stan Foster took the east and did a phenomenal job. I took the central area and Nilton [Arnt] the rest. Soon Dacca was virtually free and Stan rapidly got his four eastern districts free, too. Gradually we pushed smallpox back toward the center and to the west on the border with India, and we also protected Burma. Had smallpox got to Burma, there would have been a major disaster. When Stan Music joined us in July 1973, he took over the northwest, Nilt took southwest, and from then on things went really well and we started to get on top of the problem. The disease *was* disappearing, so sure, we were optimistic, but only because we didn't known how badly off we were!

The health teams' optimism fluctuated from day to day and euphoria from hour to hour. Describing the problem as having been handed a mountain of cooked noodles and told to shift the lot using only one noodle, Dr. Stanley Music, another American epidemiologist from CDC, admits to having fantasized in his most exhausted moments how wonderful it would be if a squadron of B-47 bombers could just spray the entire country with vaccine. The military allusion is most apt, for Music, stocky, strong of build and conviction, pragmatic and direct, could easily merge into a military background. He joined on a two-year contract and was given five districts in the northwest, approximately one-quarter of the country, as well as a Land Rover, vaccine, some needles, and a driver. Eventually he was to get his own "Hell's Angels," four Bangladeshis with motorbikes. He drove northward to meet everyone assigned to help, but few had a clue as to what was going on. There was no transport, no proper surveillance, and no follow-up inspections. People in the public service were very poorly paid. Since they had families to support, most were moonlighting and few cared enough yet to insist on quality performance or whether anyone was actually doing the job. A signature on a piece of paper was enough to satisfy the bureaucracy. In addition, Music faced, as everyone did, a mentality they *had* to change, a social system that actively discouraged the reporting of disease. He describes his approach:

First, I had to find the man who was the local chief, find out what was his job, how he viewed smallpox, whom he took orders from, whom he gave orders to, and how the vaccine was distributed. I'd go right down the chain until I got to the bottom. In the meantime, I was looking for smallpox and kept finding it. So then I'd go to the sanitary inspector in charge of that small district and say "*Sharam*, there's smallpox in this little village about three miles from here." "Oh, really?" he would reply. "But I have a report from my worker who was there yesterday and he reports none. See, here it is, signed. This is his statement." So then I'd say, "Well, he missed it. It sure is there now. So what are you going to do?" "Well, I'll vaccinate." "How much vaccine do you have?" "None." "How do you get it?" And so step by step we would go through all the procedures and from time to time I would come back and count the remaining doses to see whether he was using the vaccine. They thought this most unfair.

And so we progressed, by imposing stresses and strains and interventions and by facilitating things that otherwise would have taken an inordinate amount of time. It would have been best to educate the locals to do the job themselves, but the situation was so bad that I couldn't be an adviser, and only tell the Bengalis what to do, and still expect smallpox to be eradicated in my lifetime.

There was nothing glamorous or romantic about the lives of those in the field. From their homes in Dacca they went to the deep countryside for twenty-five days, rarely washing properly, sleeping where they could, eating well if they adapted to local food, subjecting themselves to enormous physiological stress if they didn't. Dysentery was a permanent feature of their lives in either case. Many were in Asia for the first time, some had never left their own countries before. They had no music, newspapers, or company, no one from a familiar background or culture, few people who spoke their language. The only intimate touch was the voice on the radio from smallpox headquarters in Dacca. They would be drenched to the skin or suffocating in high temperatures and higher humidities. They had to adapt, they had to understand, they had to be patient, and they had to complete each job, however long it took, however distant the place.

They did some things of which they are still ashamed, others of which they are still proud. Music says,

In Bangladesh, I got as close to assault as I would ever care to get. I broke into a man's house and vaccinated him and his family against his repeated objections.

He took me to court and the magistrate threw out the case. He [the plaintiff] *should* have won, but in their system he had no recourse. If a Bangladeshi had done that to a man, he would have been really clobbered. In another instance, a Bengali physician, my friend, physically intervened with his body to take a blow aimed at me, for I had exceeded the bounds of propriety.

But later, as we learned and so changed our methods we didn't have these frustrated responses. Yet we had to demonstrate that there could be no exceptions. So even though, emotionally, these were some of my worst moments they were also some of my best ones, too, because they were the breaking point, when the realization finally dawned on everyone that something different *had* to be done, for the system in place was quite inadequate to eradicate smallpox. If my brief anger accomplished that – fine. But I recognized afterward that anger could not be the way to perform the job. There had to be a different way and so we all began to look for alternatives.

Although each individual's recollections of these first two years contain elements similar to Music's, others are highly personal and some contain elements of farce. When Geoff Taylor found smallpox at one location in Dacca, Nick Ward confirmed the outbreak, then posted guards at the entrance to take the names and addresses of everyone entering or leaving. Soon the guards had nothing to do. The building housed what was probably the only brothel in Bangladesh, and since no one wanted to be identified, the house's takings dropped 95 percent over the ten days of the infectious period.

Other experiences were more dramatic. The Frenchman, Dr. Daniel Tarantola, small, vital, blue-eyed, and handsome, brought a professional competence and mischievous Gallic humor to his work. Employed by a French charity, "Brothers to All Men," he was recruited to Bangladesh in 1973, by Stan Foster. His English was poor: lacking grammar, syntax, and vocabulary, he could understand only 10 percent of what Stan Foster said. His Bengali was a little better but at least he could talk with his area coordinator, Stan Music, who spoke French fluently. In the end the foreigners invented "smallpox Bengali," a pidgin with a vocabulary of some 400 words.

Tarantola was posted to the far north, and when he arrived in Dinajpur armed with a two-way radio, he found no one knew anything about him. He finally contacted smallpox headquarters in Dacca, but since he kept on saying, "Who am I?" instead of "Who are you?" Dacca headquarters staff was baffled. Then light dawned: "You are Mobile 3," he was told, and from then on the radio operator always knew when it was Mobile 3 calling, since he announced himself by saying, "This is Super

Frog." His humor may have surfaced quickly, but soon he was submerged by the Everest dimensions of his job.

Dr. Tarantola's world was watery – the tributaries, the backwaters, the banks, and the sand islands called *chars* – of the Brahmaputra. In speedboats he would chase the sailing vessels up the main channel. In simple, curved river ferries that ploughed backward and forward between the banks, poled from the stern, he would be eased into the backwaters to find people eking out their lives on sandbanks or in small inlets. Exquisitely beautiful in the dry season and in spring, when the green of the rice fields rested the eyes and the brilliant red of the cotton trees stood out as a vivid counterpoint, his world turned murky and dangerous in the humid monsoon summer. The water rose at tremendous speeds, yielding up spitting cobras and writhing pythons onto the muddy banks as they, and the people, tried to escape the floods. As the levels mounted the *chars* would become submerged and his patients would move; as the river changed course a settlement he was monitoring would be swept away in the freshet and the people with it. The beauty was quite literally skin deep; the rivers were lethal, full of cholera and other infections.

Some recollections still pain Tarantola.

My saddest time came in Kurigram in North Rangput district, with an outbreak in ten villages where people had been most helpful. They always called us in early, gave good reports and identified all contacts. Well, my team visited the villages and vaccinated with the only vaccine on hand – an imported brand donated from a developed country – but suspected of not being very good. We went back a few days later to see if the vaccine had taken, and I was very surprised to see that many shots had not. So I radioed Dacca for more vaccine and we did everyone again. Then I saw a twelve-year-old boy sitting on a heap of hay, crying. "Why are you crying?" I asked. "I'm afraid of dying," he replied. "But why would you die? You've been vaccinated?" "Yes, but I know I'm getting smallpox, exactly as that man there is." He was right: he died a week later.

Other experiences are recalled with quiet pleasure. Where the Brahmaputra forms the border with India, the river is very wide and, each year as the floodwaters recede, the *chars* reemerge from the stream. Empty and lonely places, these sandbanks provide isolated shelter and are well-known places of refuge. Tarantola had checkposts at every single river crossing and local guards on each ferry, literate and educated people who, because of high unemployment, were glad to have a job. Early one evening he was in the *dak* bungalow at Sundarganj in Rangpur district, when a report came in: someone with smallpox had crossed on the ferry, his face carefully hidden. It was thought to be a notorious murderer, Robibar (the name means "Sunday"), who had gone to his hut on a remote *char* in midriver. The guards had not dared intervene, for he was notoriously violent and was accompanied by his personal bodyguard of five strong men.

Feeling that some protection might be called for, Tarantola went first to the local police station. On hearing his request, the chief turned to his colleague and said, "What is the size of our forces?"

"Two."

He turned back to Tarantola: "Then I can't give you two men, for one must always man the station. I can't give you one man either, for the rules say a soldier cannot go without the chief, and a chief cannot go without a subordinate. So no one can go."

Tarantola said he appreciated the dilemma and he'd go alone. Buf if he never returned, would they please inform Dacca, the French Embassy, WHO, and the United Nations? The policeman decided that the rules could, perhaps, be bent a little, so they all set off on bicycles, with some food wrapped in cloth tied around their waists. They had to cross four subsidiary rivers on four different ferries to get to the main channel, but by one o'clock in the morning were in the area where Robibar was hidden. They left the bikes and started to walk. Tarantola recalls:

It was a full moon, and the light was superb, crystal cold, and so beautiful. The sand from the rivers is full of silica and sparkles under the moonlight. We were on the alert though, constantly startled by the noises of the night, because we were in an area known to be frequented by many criminals.

We walked for two hours. As we waded out to the *char*, sometime around 3:00 A.M., the smallpox guards pointed out the hut. We could see a light inside. People were hanging around and my guards refused to go farther. The two policemen had long since disappeared. I went on alone, carrying my white hat in my hand so they could see me, and while I was still 100 yards away, started to talk: "I'm not a policeman. I'm not a soldier. Look, I'm a foreign doctor. I've come to help. There are no policemen with me. Please don't worry."

I saw someone come to the doorway with a long object in his hands and I knew it was a gun. I wasn't particularly courageous – in fact I was terrified – but I had no choice. Running away would have made me a good target, so I kept walking and talking. Robibar stepped forward as I came up and I saw that all he had in his hands was a bench. He put it on the ground and said, "Please sit down. Will you drink tea with me?"

After drinking tea, Tarantola vaccinated Robibar and his body-guards. But the man was desperate: he knew he was going to die and he wanted to return to his mother's house in his home village. He had already traveled for miles and had only a few more to go on what was clearly his last journey. His insistent pleading was agonized but Tarantola didn't see how he could possibly agree. He tried to explain about the disease, the inoculation campaign, and the need to keep him isolated. Under the clear, cold moon, the confrontation was drawn-out and tense but finally, Tarantola agreed to take him home.

They rested till dawn, then put Robibar on a stretcher, and the small procession walked for five hours. Ahead went outriders like those in medieval times who would warn people: "Stay back: the pox is coming." Twenty others surrounded the stretcher in a protective cordon and vaccinated anyone who approached. The village had already been alerted by radio, a messenger sent ahead, and by the time the sick man arrived, every single inhabitant had been vaccinated. Robibar was taken straight to his mother's house where, two days later, he died.

The compassion and humanity of the teams showed itself at every turn. Yet from time to time, most foreigners exceeded the bounds of propriety, all sorts of bounds and all sorts of proprieties. During one period the military commandeered all the gasoline. It was vital that the surveillance teams be kept mobile, and each leader was determined that *his* was not going to go short. The methods of obtaining gasoline varied from buying it legally, to buying it on the black market with a kickback to a local person to store it, to stealing it. Once, in the middle of a Bangladesh night, two foreigners and four Bengalis executed a neat commando operation. They located a freight train in a siding with one tanker car full of gasoline. About one o'clock in the morning, they decoupled the train, dragged the car out, and between then and sunrise, emptied as much gasoline as they could into five-gallon cans. Then they pushed the car back into position and vanished into the night.

Other problems generated other solutions. One year at harvest time, just after a famine, labor was short because people were gathering in the harvest. Not only were the harvesters paid fifteen *takas* – about eight cents – a day, but they could stuff handfuls of rice into their clothes as well. The daily pay of the surveillance teams was only ten *takas*. Their leaders wanted to match the harvest rate, but the bureaucrats refused on the grounds that to do so would feed inflation and since the harvest had priority, the health workers might leave temporarily to gather it in no matter how much they were paid. Once more a variety of imaginative solutions evolved, from hiring a few workers who didn't exist and drawing their pay, to one that required the most careful covering. A few smallpox outbreaks were invented in nonexistent villages, forms filled out characterizing them, fictional workers indented for coping with them, cash authorized to underwrite them. The money thus acquired was used to increase the pay of the teams to the harvesters' level. There are now, it is said, some learned papers written by some very learned people, that discuss some very puzzling epidemiologic patterns of smallpox in the last stages of the campaign of a form never seen before in the history of this disease.

The foreigners lived a schizophrenic existence. Once a month they returned to Dacca to recuperate, in theory at least. Dropping from irritation and frustration, emotionally and physically exhausted, they would take a bath, have several drinks, then go to headquarters, to give their reports and attend meetings. Held in a shabby, bare room in a long prefabricated building called the "submarine," these meetings were not the cool, objective discussions of calm scientists. They were emotional, fiery, argumentative battles over tactics, methods, difficulties, supplies, and ethics, and they sometimes lasted through the night.

Elsewhere in Dacca, they faced different sorts of troubles. Bureaucracy, both WHO's and that of Bangladesh, was one. In each the unwavering principle was the same: Don't rock the boat. But there were worse problems. One foreign WHO representative, compulsive and almost psychotic, regularly caused administrative and personal havoc. A local Bengali health minister frequently telephoned in the middle of the night, calling out exhausted people to interminable meetings where he would pontificate for hours. Obliged to attend at least a few diplomatic parties, they would be given champagne and hear shocked people say, aghast: "Do you really mean to say out there they eat with their hands?"

They would come to the city to rest, only to find themselves caught up in a new round of exhausting activities. The tensions were constant and their disputes, though minor, understandable. They had to unwind somehow: they took their stress out on anybody they could, most often their wives.

The wives kept open house and here the men would congregate, always troubled in mind: Were they doing things the right way? Should they allow people to be woken up by a needle in the arm? Was it appropriate to offer rewards for reporting smallpox, for did this not undermine the proper tradition of health work? They were not people who were quick to complain, but by the end of 1973, the exigencies of a stressful life in a poverty-stricken country had eroded their natural buoyancy. Two years after a civil war meant two years into a new set of corruptions and they were still battling with extreme weather, with ferries that didn't come, cars

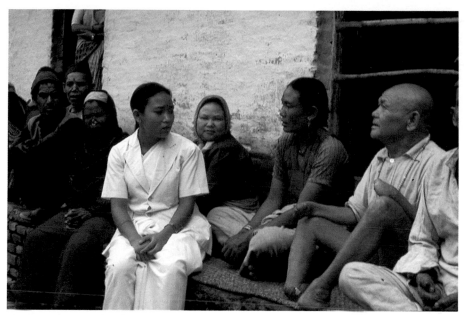

Not everyone catches leprosy. The nurse is the daughter of the man on the right. Born in the leprosarium, she has lived surrounded by leprosy, yet remains leprosy-free. (David Collison)

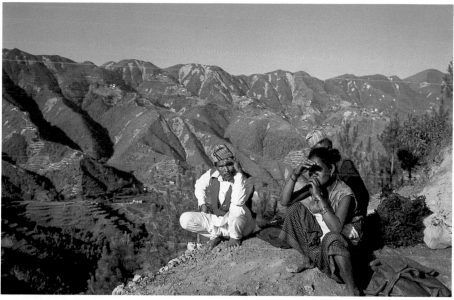

To reach patients, one must cross rough terrain. (David Collison)

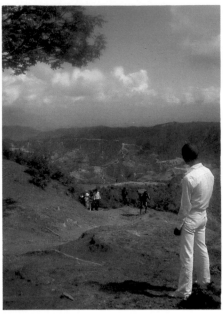

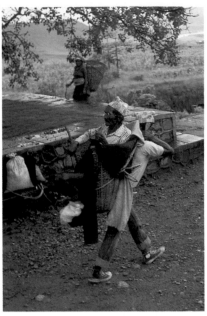

Bisha, the parademic, waits for his colleagues to reach the top of the pass.
(David Collison)

A leprosy victim is being carried to the clinic. (David Collison)

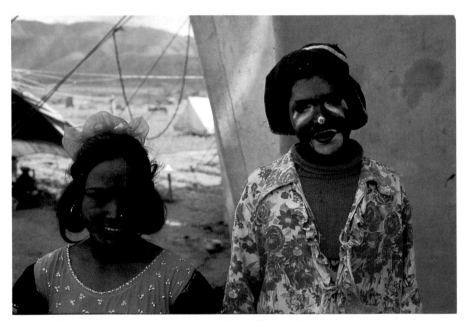

Well and happy, Rameysh the clown and his wife pose for their picture.
(Michael Johnstone)

Quest for the Killers

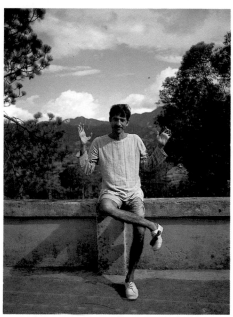

A proud Bhim Prasad shows off his recon-structed hand. (Michael Johnstone)

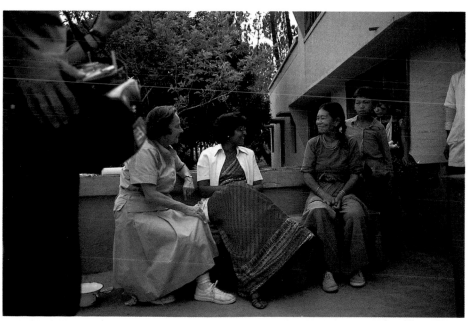

Shanta Maya, with her son Shaila, tells her story to Dr. Susie Samuels and the author. (Michael Johnstone)

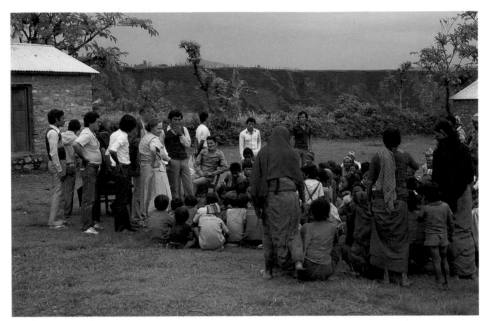

A village meeting on leprosy control; parademics and the author are on the left.
(Michael Johnstone)

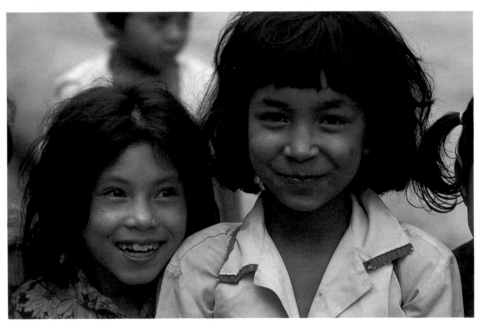

These children, or their parents, may be the last outcasts.
(David Collison)

Quest for the Killers

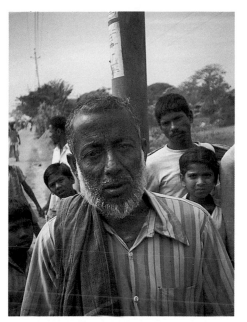

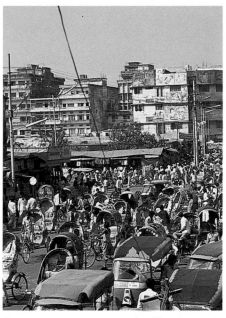

Victim of smallpox. (Alan Patient)   *Dacca is a teeming capital. (Alan Patient)*

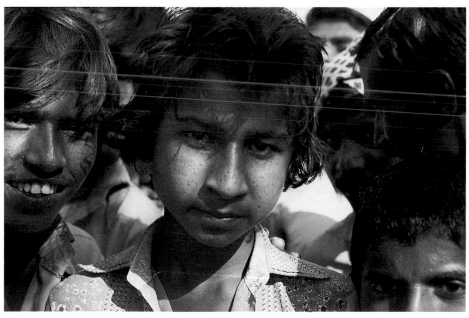

Victims of smallpox. (Alan Patient)

Quest for the Killers

Karwan bazaar where smallpox raged. (Alan Patient)

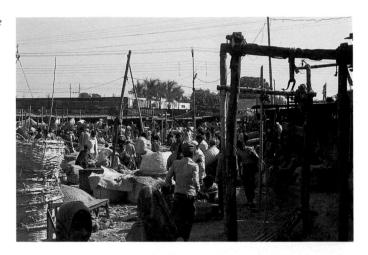

Lewis Kaplan and Nick Ward in Karwan bazaar. (Alan Patient)

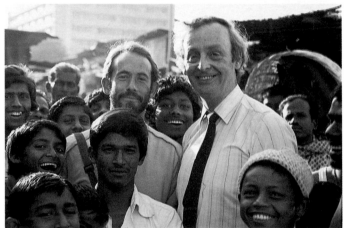

Every dwelling had to be checked for small-pox. (Alan Patient)

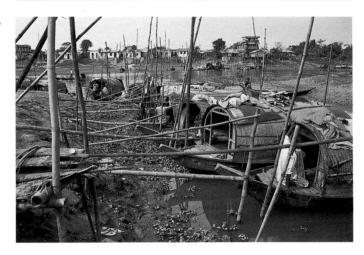

Quest for the Killers

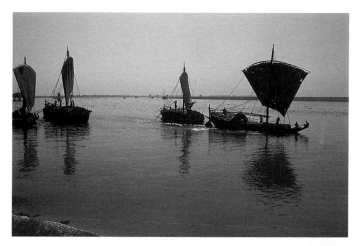

The virus traveled down the river. (Alan Patient)

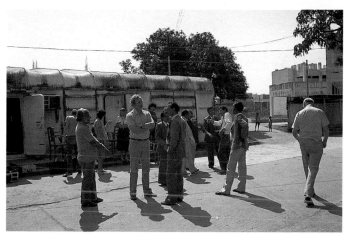

The doctors relax outside the "Submarine" headquarters. (Alan Patient)

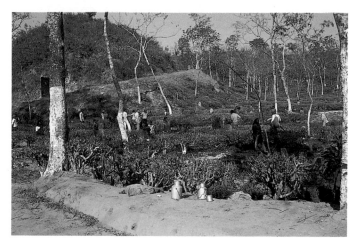

Tea pickers in Sylhet. (Alan Patient)

Quest for the Killers

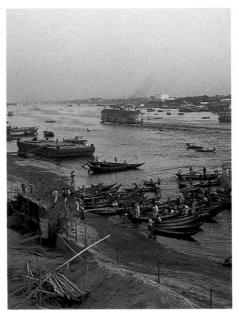

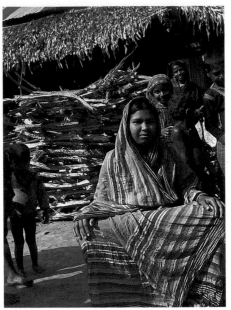

The "Speedy Rocket" leaves for Bhola Island. (Alan Patient)

Bilkisunessa, eleven years old, led the
health workers to Rahima Banu on Bhola
Island. (Alan Patient)

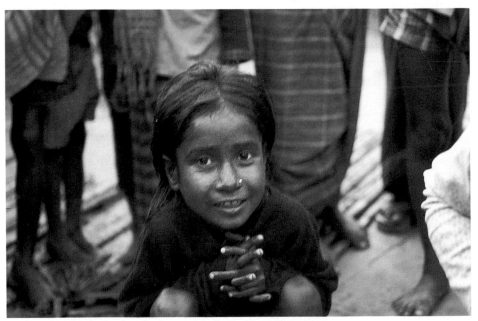

Rahima Banu, the last victim of Variola major in the world.
(Alan Patient)

Quest for the Killers

that broke down, food that ran out. Worse, whether in the city or in the countryside, the one thing they had all to live with was the total absence of privacy. Crowds of people would gather, to stare and stare and stare – and never stop. "It was easy," Daniel Tarantola comments, "to be driven insane by this. One needed the most enormous self-control because, in the end, you know, it becomes just more than curiosity – eventually there's a sadistic element within it. In a way, you can't blame them, but once they realize that it's getting to you they intensify their attention, stare unyieldingly, and if you're not careful, it can turn into a contest of wills."

Nick Ward describes the contrasts:

The people at headquarters in Dacca had a fairly ordered kind of life. They could even get the odd drink and have a circle of like-minded friends. The rest of us, myself included, would come in at the end of the month and do one of two things: either drink yourself silly or go off for a rest and recuperation that didn't really exist. You might even freak out for a bit, without much contact with colleagues, and then go back into the field. But what usually happened was that others would come and sleep on your floor for they did not particularly want to go to the hotels, so when you got up in the morning there tended to be all sorts of people around. Our houses were always open to the people in the field – the Americans were particularly good at this. We would rustle up a couple of bottles of gin and people would come in for a party. But it would be smallpox people and a smallpox party.

Our conversations were incredibly boring – what you had done about this month's outbreak and what you planned to do next month. We were the *biggest* bores. People tended to ask us to parties once but never again, for you would have a smallpox enclave sitting around on the floor, talking about patterns of transmissions here and what had to be done there. They could not understand, I think, why this strange group did not want to talk to other people but only to each other.

It was tremendously hard on families. It was smallpox all the time to the complete exclusion of everything else. Our wives were incredibly neglected: there was no time to be sensitive to their needs. If one had to draw up a balance sheet, they were very much second choice to smallpox, and marriages were subjected to the most enormous strains. I think that they were a remarkable group of women and their contribution has never been adequately recognized.

Nevertheless they all still recall those years as a magnificent experience in which they were privileged to participate.

It was wonderful in a variety of ways [Ward goes on]. The program may have spoiled our social life and wrecked our family life, but our personal lives had real purpose.

But perhaps just as important was that with its superb leadership, the program provided a high degree of team spirit and this made people become committed as much to other people as to the job.

You must absolutely realize that this was not a matter of good luck. It was good management which started when D.A. [Donald Henderson] was himself appointed [as program director]. He then set about defining exactly what needed to be done to get rid of this disease, and if this meant breaking established WHO rules, then they were broken and they were broken to the benefit of the people in the field. But the most important thing that he did was to make absolutely sure that the people selected were the right people for the job and not just people who were politically acceptable to a world organization. In addition, D.A. is a very charismatic individual. He is personable, friendly to people who are vastly his junior. He cares for them.

But, by the end of 1973, and two years into their campaign, the blazing fires of wild optimism were being quenched by cold realism. Despite all their efforts they weren't winning. They actually knew a mere 45 percent of all existing cases and though this was more than four times greater than the previous year, it was nowhere near enough. Two things then changed, the leadership and the structure of the system.

As head of the program in Bangladesh, Ward had carried the greatest burden. He had to combat massive epidemics with a small staff, no supplies, and little money. When the money ran out he used his own. When support seemed to be ebbing, he searched for patrons. Ruefully he recalls an occasion when he made three minor requests to the British High Commission and had an exquisitely polite, but very firm, refusal, to everyone. By contrast Stan Foster arrived with full backing from CDC in Atlanta. Were more people, money, and supplies needed? He had the green light to go ahead and order them. Armed with field experience, American know-how and firm back-up support, he saw deficiencies in both the tactical plan and its execution, and promptly told Ward so.

Everyone loved, and still loves, Nick Ward. As Tarantola told me, "Nick hates quarrels and he never revealed the extent of the disagreement between him and Foster. Had he done so, the team would have split and taken sides." Willingly, happily, and, above all, quietly, Nick Ward handed the reins over to Stan Foster, and left Bangladesh. "It was," he now says, "absolutely the right thing to do," for Foster, he insists, was a brilliant, international professional, compared to whom he, Ward, was only an amateur.

Stan Foster does not agree:

Nick was marvelous, a very hard worker, one of the best fieldworkers and the most sensitive person I have ever seen. He was just *good* and when I felt that we had organizational problems, I told Nick and he quit on the spot. He felt it as a criticism and it was really a tremendous personal blow. He left Bangladesh somewhat scarred, perhaps never wanting to return. But he didn't "quit" in the normal sense of the term, for whenever I'd get into trouble, which was just about every three months, I'd call and say, "Nick, can you come?" and he always came. He was what we needed: he knew Dacca better than anybody else; he had excellent relationships with the people here and he trusted everybody to do their work properly; he was an incredibly good leader. There is a difference between a leader and a director. I was just a director.

The second change also concerned Nick Ward. Shortly before leaving, he called on the Secretary of Health of Bangladesh to make what he now says was his single most important contribution to the campaign. The health service was in the process of being restructured and each existing worker would now become a family health worker trained to do six basic procedures, including smallpox vaccination. In addition, twelve thousand more would be recruited. Ward said to the Secretary, "This is going to be very good indeed for Bangladesh in the future. But for *now*, would you please let us have twenty-five special teams to carry out smallpox surveillance, so our program will be able to continue?"

They were given their teams and for leaders chose the twenty-five best Bangladeshis they knew. Backed by firm government support, the teams worked phenomenally well. The smallpox workers received extra training in epidemiology and were paid extra money. Although they were taken out of the ordinary career hierarchy, many of them were given highly responsible positions afterward, for they were recognized as being the most energetic and competent people in the country. Foster posted each one to districts other than their own, as "foreigners," where, armed with initiative, incentives, and status they quickly spotted the gaps and streamlined the work. They were the true intermediaries between the administrators in Dacca and those crucial local officers at the periphery, and they knew how to channel resources through the jungles of bureaucracy, personal pride, vanity, and greed.

As the new director, Stan Foster had a vital hand in this restructuring. Two separate government divisions – the malaria bureau and the government health service – dealt with health and in both there had been too much busywork, paper pushing, and too much buck passing. Says Foster,

When we identified this as a problem, the government promptly said: "Well, what would *you* do? So one night we sat down and came up with a plan for a single structure for smallpox from the bottom to the top. For each small district, there was a smallpox officer, then another above for the subdivision, then one for each major district and so on. I nearly made the mistake of choosing the people, but then I realized that if we were giving the local district people the responsibility for the work, we should also give them the responsibility of finding the best people to do it.

Then we introduced a reward system for reporting. We introduced just a single reward but the health workers were worried that the public would claim it all. So they kept silent and only a few people knew about its existence. But when we doubled the sum and divided the money between the first person to report the case and the first health worker to confirm it, the public quickly learned about the reward.

Some foreigners were unhappy about all this, seeing a reward as an unnecessary "capitalist" gloss on the program; others were unhappy about the overtime allowances paid to the team's local staff, whose load had increased from an original five hours a day to as much as twenty. For when the campaign ended and the financial rewards slumped, would their enthusiasm for health programs also slump? Only one thing about rewards ever worried Stan Foster. There was so much smallpox in Bangladesh that the reward for reporting a case was six dollars. But across the border in India, now practically smallpox-free, the reward had risen to nearly five hundred dollars; he was afraid that patients would be spirited over, but they never were.

New techniques to spread the word were being tried everywhere in Asia. In India, where a tribal group in Bihar was demonstrating its skepticism for the nth time, Larry Brilliant promised: "In a minute an aircraft will come over and drop an important message." It did, in the form of thousands of fluttering leaflets that read: "Have you seen anyone looking like this?" In Bangladesh, they mobilized an elephant. The Bengali health leader in charge of Dacca city realized that if a slogan was painted on an elephant's side and it was walked around for a couple of days, huge crowds would be attracted, for the animal was rare in the country. Large posters are widely used in Asia to advertise films, so the elephant carried two vast ones on its sides, with the message "Have you seen . . . ?" painted in red, white, and blue.

Fresh approaches also were applied to the management of the teams. Stan Foster describes some:

From time to time, we would give all our workers a total picture of the global campaign, as well as in Bangladesh, but then we'd focus in and spend a great deal of time explaining why house searches were necessary. I would select 1,500 villages at random, to be checked by various district officers and as people began to realize their work was being checked, the quality of their searches improved.

Our very first, nationwide, house search picked up 108 new outbreaks and the incidence began to go down. By looking for *all* rash cases next, we increased the sensitivity of the search and in the next series we picked up 40,000 new rashes. Not all were smallpox but some were. By the end of the campaign, in some of our best searches, we could so mobilize our people that 89 percent of *all* the houses in the country would be visited. Each worker was allocated 1,000 houses. Some worked hard, some did nothing, but even so, roughly *twelve million houses would be covered in seven to nine days.* So as the years rolled by, our procedure evolved, from surveillance teams alone in market and school searches, to the single reward system, to the coopting of the 12,000 workers into the health system, to the double reward, to detailed house-to-house searching. And as this evolved, so too did other, crucially important things, those that related to the people's perceptions of smallpox. There was a gradual change of attitude. The government was seen to be doing something, so the people responded, for it was now worthwhile to respond. And this change was reflected in our data: 40 to 45 percent of the last 119 outbreaks were voluntarily reported by the public.

Slowly their grasp tightened yet again and they refined their techniques still further. An overnight stay in the villages now became mandatory so that people could be vaccinated either late at night, or early in the morning before they'd left for work or school. Foster recalls:

When we made that change we became more accepted and that helped. Going from house to house, with somebody from the village to help, I'd vaccinate, often at night. There might be eight kids lying on the bed and we'd vaccinate them before they woke up. But still we were working twenty hours a day, seven days a week, twenty-eight days a month, and occasionally one lost one's temper. On the whole, though, we found that when we had insisted that a family be vaccinated, they would end up laughing and help us to do the house next door. Once they realized that we were not going to hurt them, then they would come onto our side very strongly.

Though the total number of people vaccinated increased, the methods were still not good enough, and the program's leaders needed to find the reason why. Their final strategy was one that developed solely by systematically analyzing their *failures* and the plan that evolved as a result of this critical analysis, had four elements: (1) isolate patients in their own houses; (2) post two guards day and night; (3) list, find, and vaccinate everyone within a half mile; (4) search a two-mile area around for all other cases.

The goal they now set was that no outbreak should produce any new cases after the incubation period of two weeks, and they regularly checked to see how many workers met that goal. Stan Foster recalls one brilliant Bengali who told him: "We have a problem. We are doing everything the books say and still we are not stopping smallpox." Then, with a big smile, he went on: "But today I found out why. When we find a case, we have been asking for a list of visitors, but they are not giving us the names of relatives, for they don't consider them to be visitors." From then on all relatives were regarded as face-to-face contacts and were vaccinated even if they'd not been near their infectious kin. Thus the final tactics developed out of problem-solving of this kind.

Though a new wave of optimism spread among the teams there were still maddening frustrations. Nick Ward recalls a recurring one:

It was nearly always the educated and the rich who were difficult. The poor and the humble were no trouble at all. I remember when I was down to the last known outbreak in Dacca city. There'd been a slight mistake over one mild case we'd put down as chicken pox. The patient had only half-a-dozen spots, but since he had been walking around for a number of days, we had to be sure that there were no more cases. So I was checking a block of flats owned by senior civil servants and I rang at the door of one smart place and a man answered. "No," he said, "we've got no smallpox here. There is no need for you to come in." But I insisted: "Could I please see your family?" Eventually, I pushed into the flat and into the bathroom. There, cowering in the bath, was his daughter, covered with smallpox. Now this man was a senior government civil servant – intelligent, rich, and influential – but he didn't want his daughter taken to the hospital. It was this kind of thing that used to drive one mad.

But look at the good side of it all, the gentleness and the niceness of the average Bangladeshi. He's not a person with a big ego. He's kind, humble, and anxious to please. He's got nothing at all in his house, but what little he has he will always share with you. Another good thing was the commitment of our teams. Once they knew you were looking after them they would do quite incredibly good work and you had their absolute loyalty. Our relationship with them was marvelous – a mutual confidence and a respect for each other's judgment. We give them *all* the credit for, unlike most of the people in the health structure at that time, you could turn your back and still work went on at a high level.

"We were learning from them all the time," says Stan Foster on this same point.

It took me a year to recognize the value of regular debriefings, but when people left or were reassigned, they came up with the truth: where the problems were, who was hiding cases, who was stealing money. When we found we were missing houses, the Bangladeshis drew maps for us. When we were missing people, they made up books to list everyone. They told us that patients were hungry and going out foraging, so we provided money for food. They told us that people had to move once to harvest their rice and again to sell it, so we paid patients a daily wage to stay in isolation. They told us that one house guard would fall asleep or run away, so we always had two; that the supervisors would not sleep in the village for they had nothing to eat, so we recruited village people into the program who provided food for the teams. In the end, they could train the locals in half an hour flat and then get a 95 to 98 percent effective vaccination in their village. It was quite incredible. What might be difficult for others to understand is that all these things were done essentially by people who had barely any primary education.

By June 1974 the program knew 53 percent of all cases occurring and the number of new ones was dropping fast. In August there was a meeting in Delhi where everyone was asked to give estimates of when smallpox would be gone. When the leader of the Indian campaign said the spring of 1975, everyone laughed. It was much too cautious: they could do better than that. As for Bangladesh, Foster said that they would bid farewell to smallpox, forever, by November 1974.

A debate now developed between Foster and his staff, who felt that since all the eighty-nine remaining foci of smallpox had been now identified, eighty-nine professional epidemiologists should be brought in, one to cover each outbreak and smother every case as it erupted. Foster said no. He wanted to keep the teams small, for he felt their closeness and understanding lay at the heart of the program's success. By October 1974, there were *still* only eighty-nine infected villages and the exact location of every outbreak was known. Foster now publicly predicted that smallpox would be eradicated by December.

When the monsoon finally ended in August 1974, the floods came late but instead of retreating, the water stayed high. The Brahmaputra burst its banks right across the area of the eighty-nine infected villages and tens of thousands of people scattered to high ground, their homes under water, their crops wiped out. As famine began to stalk the land, a massive tide of people began to move. The first city they swamped was Mymensingh in the north, where every night thousands slept on the railway platforms before moving on to Jaimalpur. Each morning, Nick Ward had healthworkers go round and lift the blankets to see who was still alive, who had smallpox, and to vaccinate quietly. The situation was bad certainly, yet if smallpox had stayed in the north it could have been contained. But these were desperate people and they wanted food, not vaccination, so they went to Dacca.

The next six months were an unrelenting and all consuming nightmare, especially for Stan Foster. Ten days before Christmas, his son became critically ill with a spinal tumor and the Fosters feared he would never walk again. Foster's wife took the boy to the States for surgery and stayed with him for the next two-and-a-half months. Then, in January 1975, smallpox erupted in Dacca.

One rural case had been confirmed, but Dacca seemed to be the source, and if it *was*, they were in for another major epidemic. So the most intensive search possible was mounted, but no one could discover smallpox. So once again, Foster telephoned Ward. He was at the Imperial Hotel, Delhi, when the message arrived, having a farewell party with two old friends, epidemiologists. All three caught the next plane to Bangladesh.

I remember the day I got back clearly [Ward says]. I went straight to the area where the cases were suspected – Karwan bazaar. My one conceit was that I knew Dacca city vastly better than any other foreigner, perhaps better than any other foreigner ever had. It didn't take very long to find five cases. They were in the market and if you looked at the area superficially, it seemed just a small slum. But, in fact, the shanties, just pieces of bamboo matting leant up against the walls, flowed back behind the railway in a myriad of little alleys. The smallpox was right in there.

Then one day in February, I turned up for the usual routine examination and there were bulldozers knocking down the shanties on the order of the President, Sheik Mujibur Rahman, as part of his policy to beautify the city. This *basti* area on the airport road was the first thing visitors saw when they arrived, so it was to be bulldozed flat. I got very angry. I said, "Look, I will go and get an order. This *basti* has to stay for another two weeks, then you can do what you like with it." The chap in charge said, "Yes, I understand what you are doing."

It took me about four hours to get action at the diplomatic level. When I returned the bulldozers were again knocking things down and this time I really flipped my lid. I nearly wept. I got hold – again, almost physically – of the commanding officer. I put him in my Land Rover and drove around to see the President. As we drove through the gates I said to the guards, "It's all right, we are going to see the Sheik," and walked straight into his office. Fortunately, he was off to the airport to meet someone or I would have certainly been thrown out of the country.

So I left and cooled off, realizing that I was going to get myself into political hot water. By now it was about seven o'clock at night and many of our people from the field were in the city for the end-of-the-month get-together. So we all piled everyone into Land Rovers, and went back to the *basti* but we were much too late. Most people had gone.

In the next two weeks we had 180 smallpox outbreaks scattered all over the city and *all* could be traced back to the *basti*. Once more, this allowed the whole of Bangladesh to become reinfected again, by the same centrifuge effect, and this was when we became really discouraged – but I was more angry than anything.

Suddenly, with India and the rest of the world near zero, Bangladesh exploded right back to its worst point ever. The period from January to October 1975 was, for an anxious Donald Henderson, the worst time of any in the global campaign. Bangladesh looked like being the country on whose rocks the campaign would founder and, as Henderson well knew, many people were ready to say, "We told you so." The country had always been regarded as the cradle of recurring cholera epidemics, and over and over he had heard the refrain: "It's going to be the same. You'll never eradicate smallpox in Bangladesh." The government was in turmoil, refugees were all over the place, relief agencies were trying to get reestablished, and the teams were back to square one.

Foster's depression spiraled downward: everything seemed to be conspiring against them. Torn by thoughts of failure and anxiety about his son, his personal agony intensified. Along with his colleagues, he longed for the end of spring, for the annual moment when the peak would pass and the figures start going down. The end of spring came, but the figures didn't budge. In January, he had written to Henderson, "If these floods continue, all hell will break loose"; in February, the *bastis* were destroyed, and his wife and children were still away. March was a terrible month. The figures remained high. Reverend John McKinley, a Baptist missionary and a dear friend, recalls kidding Foster, saying, "You'll be famous," and realized what a dreadful mistake he had made when he heard the bitter rejoinder, "I'll be infamous." In that month, too, the psychotic WHO representative finally had to be pulled out; in addition Foster was under constant pressure from the Ministry of Health, from local officials, even from his own superiors at the CDC. Perhaps the selective strategy was wrong for a place like Bangladesh; perhaps only mass vaccination would do.

In three months matters had gone from bad to worse to appalling, and at this point, Foster confesses he became totally disabled. All remember his agony with sympathy, all recall the same vignette of his distress. He would go to one house, dazed as if concussed, sit down, say nothing, then, after a long pause, only "Do you think we can make it?" shake his head, leave, go to another house, and repeat the scene.

Whatever effectiveness I had [Foster says], came from other people's support. There was no backbiting, no condemnations. I was carried by my staff and my wife and without them I would have completely folded. Rangara, an Indian physician, was always optimistic, always buoyed me up. It was his military training. Convinced optimism, he reminded me, had been the secret of survival during the military campaign in the jungles of Burma in World War II. "Never give up," he'd say. "You'll do it."

Finally the situation was so terrible we had to declare a national emergency and mobilize additional resources. The Swedish government was magnificent: they came through with $25 million immediately. I picked up the phone and said to D. A., "I need you." One of the reasons the program succeeded is that whenever we said that, D. A. came. He came to persuade the government that this really was an emergency situation and, since India was free [of smallpox], if they didn't buckle down and tackle the problem, there was a real chance that Bangladesh would be quarantined.

Over and over D. A. came in and one day Foster offered his resignation. When D. A. refused to accept it, Foster confessed he would have been totally shattered had it been accepted. But he also realized that, if he was to recover his effectiveness, he must leave for a while, so he asked Daniel Tarantola to take over as acting leader, then departed for three months. Tarantola felt Nick Ward really should have the job but characteristically Ward didn't mind one bit. Tarantola now says:

There wasn't really very much to do except sign the forms, for by then the team leaders were so good they didn't really need anyone at the top. But I must admit that the situation had caught us by surprise because I suspect we'd become a little overconfident. We'd made no provision for natural disasters so we had no reserves, nor additional staff. We had, in fact, begun demobilizing people. Now we realized that we would break transmission only if we found ways to move faster than the people, who were still moving all over the place. This was the key. We mobilized teams who would race through the country at incredible speed: if the people moved by bullock cart, we went by motorbike; by bus, then we used Land Rovers; by boats and we chased them in speedboats; by train and we placed our workers on trains, too, and radioed ahead to their destinations. For example, an epidemiologist on boat surveys heard that a sick fisherman had left Bogra the day before, going home to Barisal in the south — a trip of forty-eight hours, involving one train and two boat rides. The people knew his name, the date of his smallpox attack, and the village he was making for. By the time he arrived, the entire village had been vaccinated, guards were already in place, and he was taken straight to the isolation hut already prepared.

We also knew that community support was vital if we were to succeed, and we thought we had it. Then one day a report came in from the north that one of the local sanitary inspectors had been beaten up. We were very worried – until we learned the real reason. Some villagers had gone to report an outbreak. The men promised to go and vaccinate that day. The next day the villagers sent a messenger, emphasizing that it was urgent he come to control the outbreak. He replied that he'd come along later but never turned up. So the villages descended on him, roughed him up, took away the vaccine and vaccinated the entire village themselves. This was magnificent for it showed us not only that we had community support but that people now realized both that smallpox could be prevented and that it was not so much a gift as their right.

So once again, everyone mounted the treadmill of exhausting routine, starting work at five in the morning to continue until dark or even later, for twenty-nine days each month and the pressures built up again. Henderson recalls the time:

Talking and working with the people there, particularly during this peak time, I saw immense stress like I have never seen in all my life. There were people there who, outside of Bangladesh (I know) were perfectly fine. But under the most incredible pressures they had to endure, they came close to cracking up, psychologically. They bounced between incredible highs of joy that they were going to succeed and incredible lows of depression when they felt they never would. In spite of their unrelenting hard work and the fact that they had put their hearts and souls into the program, smallpox would suddenly explode and time after time after time, they were back to square one. Small, unforeseen things would set them back for months. The troubles they had in Bangladesh, beyond those of dealing with a government which was just assuming control, were unbelievable, and the fact that they held together as they did was a miracle. It was a real battlefield situation, and when things began to deteriorate . . . there are all sorts of quirks of personal character, or personal expectations being thwarted, so there is tension between individuals. Blame is cast; there is disappointment in the performance of others and of one's self. But if *I* ever became downcast or pessimistic, I'd only to go to Bangladesh and see them. They'd give me the courage to go back and to keep going.

Comments Nick Ward:

This worked both ways. Very few of the people sitting smugly in Geneva would come and walk the paddy fields, but D. A. did. He'd come three or four times each year, stay about five days, and there can't be many of our areas he hasn't been to. He'd attend meetings and, by talking about their individual, personal contribution to the global campaign, make our people feel that the world was watching *their* district. For us it was fun in many ways. We sat on the verandah eating rice and chicken and the children would come and listen. But D. A. must have been sick of it all, meeting after meeting after meeting, and then he would fly off to do it all over again, someplace else.

Constantly they would be reassured by the familiar stocky presence, by Henderson's booming laugh, the comfort of his arm around a shoulder, the smack of his fist into the palm of his hand as he drove home his points. Henderson himself became exhausted at times. Carol Music remembers his coming to their home, "sitting down, cooling out, listening to opera on our stereo, mesmerized. He'd just spent eight hours with the bureaucrats and the fatigue was pouring off him. They had all the time in the world but he had only two or three days to spare." And one evening he and Stan Music talked about the campaign and a way to commemorate it. There and then they created the "Order of the Bifurcated Needle," and Music took a pair of pliers, bent a needle into a zero, and D. A. took the prototype back to Geneva, where his daughter made the 1,000 copies by hand.

The situation was now so serious that the government issued an edict: anyone refusing vaccination would be imprisoned. Still more outside people had to be mobilized. Eventually there would be 12,000 local health workers and 13,000 ancillary workers, supervised by 100 foreign epidemiologists, 65 of whom came on three-month contracts. Lewis Kaplan, a student from England, was one of many "drafted" for the emergency. His parents were close friends with Henderson and while a student he was wandering around Africa when Henderson recruited him for the smallpox program. He'd already spent ten months in Ethiopia but, while waiting to go to the University of Sussex, was in Andorra, skiing, when he received a cable: *Emergency situation in Bangladesh, all experienced smallpox workers needed. Can you come?* He left immediately. His recollections, which bring this time of anxious counterattack into vivid relief, are typical of many young people thrown into the final assault.

After three days of briefing in Delhi, I arrived in Bangladesh in April 1975, just before the monsoon. The weather was awful – sticky and uncomfortable. There were nearly sixty-five foreign advisers so they took a house, the "Pox Pad," where I stayed, with room for about twenty, and anybody who was in the capital would stay there. Nick Ward asked me if I knew how to ride a motorcycle, but I didn't. So he said, "Please learn." This was on Friday. I was due to go into the field on Monday, and a Suzuki 80cc was found for me on Sunday. I went to a quiet suburban area and drove around the block several times, trying to work out which was the brake and which the clutch. I vaguely learned how to ride the thing and next day Nick took me into the field. I'd had some briefing – how to fill in the field records, how to keep the accounts, to make certain that there were four copies of every receipt. We started off in Nick's Land Rover with the two motorbikes stuck in the back. Each was heavily loaded – a mosquito net, a *huge* kit bag, four gallons of petrol, money, and a load of vaccine – everything I would need in the field.

Lewis Kaplan would be responsible for Raipura *thana,* a rural area of about 108 square miles with a population of nearly half a million people. There were no proper roads and the region was crisscrossed by rivers, one of which, the Megna, ran along the border. Twelve miles from their destination they had to abandon the Land Rover and the road for a hair-raising ride along the railroad track.

Small muddy tracks paralleled the rail lines and these were fine until one came to a bridge. In the dry season travelers simply pushed their bikes down the embankment, crossed the valley underneath the bridge, and climbed back up the other side. But this was the monsoon and the valleys were flooded. So, swearing and cursing, Lewis Kaplan learned how to lift the front wheel of the heavily laden bike onto the track first, then the back wheel, then mount and, while balancing precariously and praying fervently, move his feet along the railroad ties, and take the bike over that way. If a train did come, he was told, he should throw himself and the bike off the side as fast as he could. Sometimes people would take motor vehicles across, with two wheels balanced on one rail and the other two on the track below the opposite rail. When a huge charger of a railway engine met a small palfrey of a jeep, as it sometimes did, the one would slowly push the other back across the bridge where, more often than not, it fell over and rolled down the embankment.

There were many such bridges to cross and it took them four hours to do the final twelve miles. When they finally arrived at the main station of Methikanda, Kaplan was dehydrated and exhausted. He promptly drank gallons of water and was ready to sleep, but he had to wait in the center of the small town while Nick Ward made arrangements. Methikanda was a small place with some six food houses, a barber's shop, a couple of little stalls that sold cigarettes or biscuits, and a government *dak* bungalow where he would live. Exhausted or not, he and Ward still had to drive into the next town to meet two Bengalis from the district smallpox office. When the courtesies and formalities were over, and Kaplan had paid his respects both to the *thana* smallpox officer and his assistant health inspector, they decided he had done enough for one day. So Nick Ward briefed him a little more, hoped he'd be OK, and said he'd come back in a week or two to see if Kaplan was still functioning. Jumping on his motorbike he disappeared, leaving Kaplan very much alone. Though the *dak* bungalow was just a bedless concrete square divided diagonally in two, the young recruit collapsed on the mat and slept soundly.

The next day he called a meeting of the local health personnel, some sixty-five people employed by the government, half of whom worked on the malaria program while the others were general health workers. Some spoke English, some didn't; some were well-organized and efficient and some seemed hopelessly unable to do the tasks that fitted the job description even when there *was* a job description. His was to ensure that all members of the health service drop everything and work on the smallpox program because the number of cases had increased more than tenfold in February and March 1975, and, three months later, they were still in the middle of a major epidemic. Since Kaplan's brief had come from the Ministry of Health, everyone was very helpful except the person in charge – the *thana* health administrator, an M.B., B.S., and the only clinical doctor around. Because he was so busy he wouldn't, he said, have much to do with the smallpox program and Kaplan wasn't in a powerful enough position to force him to cooperate. Luckily his assistant was raring to get going.

Starting as he hoped to go on, Kaplan told them that he was merely a WHO adviser and that was all, for it was *their* program. But loud and clear came back the message: "We don't know what to do; you're here to help us; you alone know what's going on and you are the man with the money." As a foreigner who had been sent a long way in order to help them he *obviously* had to tell them what to do. The situation was totally different from the one he had faced in Ethiopia, where there had only been a very few health workers, where the disease had been mild, and people less bothered by it. The Ethiopians also didn't want to deal with anything coming from the outside, saying to Kaplan, "This is white man rubbish and we don't want it. Go away." In Bangladesh, by contrast, he had behind him a large bureaucratic infrastructure that was now prepared to give massive support. So together Kaplan and his new friends decided on their plan and began pulling in extra health workers for special training. Because there were so many cases and too few staff, local village people were also trained to vaccinate, but even with vaccinators and surveillance people all over the place, with the reward system and much publicity, it still wasn't enough.

Kaplan returned to Dacca in the same way and manner in which he came, and put his problem to Ward and Tarantola. They promised that whatever he needed he'd get, for he was now reporting more cases than any other district in the country. He asked for more transport first and besides his little Suzuki motorbike soon had two Honda 50's and four Chinese bicycles. These came unassembled in cardboard boxes and since no one knew how to put them together Kaplan tried himself over the next couple of days and went on trying until they worked. When the motorbikes broke down he had to fix these too. He went through three in as many months: one fell into ten feet of water, one simply collapsed, but the third was still going three months later, when his contract was up. He also had two motorboats but one never worked at all, since every time it was put in the water, it fell to pieces. The other broke down frequently but nevertheless was useful for river surveillance and bringing in supplies.

Every vehicle took a fearful pounding and getting around was hazardous. Mostly the teams rode along the little raised tracks between the paddy fields, tracks often no more than six inches wide, so they fell off again and again. Once Kaplan plunged into deep water and ended up under his bike. When he finally rose he saw about a hundred people on the bank who had materialized out of nowhere. They helped fish the bike out, but Kaplan developed a bad middle ear infection from this ducking and his hearing is still impaired.

His ignorance when he arrived matches that of Henderson's at the beginning of the campaign. "I never ever thought," he now says, "that the job would be totally impossible though if I had been more aware of what was going on perhaps I might have. But by the time I arrived in April 1975 there was a feeling from the rest of the country that we *were* getting on top of the disease. So I rode with that feeling even though I was in an outrageous situation with hundreds of fresh case reports coming in every week."

His logistic problems were formidable; at one time he was by far the largest dispenser of money in the *thana*, employing four hundred people. All he had to say was "Let it be known that I need people" and next day there would be up to a hundred to interview. When each area was declared free his staff were paid, but since at least a quarter needed paying every week, and Sunday was payday, he had to go to the bank each week and get money. He would pick up some twenty thousand *takas*, $50, in a packet of two thousand very smelly, mildewed ten-*taka* notes which the banker would count off incredibly fast. It would have taken Kaplan all day to check, so he would just believe him, shove the lot into a cardboard box tied on the back of the bike, and drive off.

Shortly after he arrived he was befriended by a local Bengali who had an air of knowing his way around. The man gave Kaplan a few timely warnings about the local politics. The two ended up by organizing the Bahini, a freedom-fighting team of young people all committed to smallpox eradication. Many other groups organized similar squads that would go out at all times of day or night.

The team of twelve would move in with megaphones. Their standard ploy would be to enter the front door and since the women would promptly rush out at the back they posted somebody at the back too, and as the people ran out to hide in the jute fields, grabbed and vaccinated them. There was one particular village on a heavily populated island in the Begna where second- and third-generation smallpox kept recurring over and over and in the end they just moved from one end of the island to the other and systematically went into every single house. People were hiding their babies in the grain bins or up on the roofs, and Kaplan felt terribly sad that he had neither time nor resources to give them health education. Like others before him, he found himself battling with conflicting emotions. He knew that there would still be resistance, no matter how much education he gave, because it was all, culturally, so alien. Yet he had to be firm, for the government was enforcing the penalty for refusal. On one occasion a surveillance team jailed two men. When Kaplan went to the prison they were on their knees begging for release. He couldn't take this at all, so asked them to go back to explain to everyone in their village why they must take vaccination. They agreed.

He made excellent use of those trains he had so feared when he crossed his first bridge. The roof was an excellent place to vaccinate and soon they established a daily routine. Climbing aboard at Methikanda, at one end of the district, they rode through to Bairhab bazaar, about twenty minutes away, just outside their district boundary. Then they'd catch the next train back through the *thana*. All day they'd be up aloft just vaccinating. They never went into the third class, because people were packed in so tight that they couldn't push through; nor into first class, because the passengers wouldn't unlock the doors. Therefore, along with the cigarette and betel-nut vendors, they'd go aloft and vaccinate the fifty people on the top of each carriage and then just jump across to the next. "It wasn't," Kaplan hastened to assure me, "quite as dangerous as it sounds, since the train was only going at thirty miles per hour and there were no tunnels."

Soon he spoke a fair amount of Bengali and adapted to the life very quickly. Within six weeks he was wearing a *lungi* with a loose shirt and eating at the one tea shop he had chosen as being slightly less unsanitary than the others. But his conditions were still very primitive. He actually slept on the cardboard boxes in which the Chinese bicycles had arrived, all piled on top of each other, for the rubber mattresses supplied were much too hot.

Once a week he'd return to Dacca. The direct route was to the southwest, but if he went north along a little trail for about two hours he could pick up the main road and then go down south to the capital. This journey was his only private time, and it was very precious. He would be very quiet, concentrating on driving and not falling off, but also reveling in the few moments of not having to deal with people. "If I went along this track *and* didn't see anyone for a quarter of a mile *and* if I was very quiet *and* coasted in on my bike *and* hid it behind a tree, I occasionally found that I could sit for the whole of fifteen minutes before someone would come along."

Before Kaplan left, his staff in Raipura gave him a huge party — as they did for everyone who came in to help. He would happily have stayed for six more months, but he had to take up his place at Sussex University. So after being debriefed by Daniel Tarantola and Nick Ward, he departed at the end of June 1975.

One month later, a completely recovered Stan Foster returned and by now the numbers were dropping fast. He had had plenty of time for reflection and with painful honesty reveals:

The whole episode taught me a lot about humility. Had we succeeded in October 1974, I would have felt it was very much my victory. Now I recognized the tremendous input and personal sacrifice of the whole WHO staff, especially Nick and Nilton. Regularly totally fed up, they just as regularly left vowing never to return. But they always did. They showed tremendous loyalty to me and the program at considerable hardship and great personal pain.

Stan Foster is a deeply religious man. Shortly after he returned, he went north to Sylhet, the region of the tea plantations, and one night while watching the sunset had a mystical experience. He was sitting quietly, quite alone, when suddenly the conviction came that they'd won. He believed he heard a voice within saying, "It's going to be all right. You're going to do it." He still was convinced that success would come even when the president, Sheik Mujibar Rahman, was assassinated in August 1975 and the specter of civil war once more rose up to haunt them. For four days, when all movement across the country stopped and the teams could not communicate with each other or even cross Dacca, they held their collective breaths. The crisis passed. By now they knew 80 percent of all occurring cases.

Suddenly, unbelievably, it was over. By mid-September the entire staff were convinced that the last case had occurred in the Chittagong; by mid-November they were sure. Six weeks went by with no fresh cases, then a cable from WHO said there would soon be a public announcement and Bangladesh would be declared free of smallpox. The press release was issued on November 14, 1975, and major newspapers like *The New York Times* ran the story. The entire staff poured into Dacca to celebrate.

The party was a very good one, full of laughter, liquor, and congratulations. Then as the stress was suddenly removed, so the tension just as suddenly snapped, neatly and cleanly, like a finely tuned string whose load has become too great. Grievances, real and imagined, swelled to the surface. Disputes that had been suppressed, personal feelings that had been ignored in the recognition that the common goal was the only thing that really mattered, erupted all at once. Arguments flared. Two Dacca administrators hammered verbally at each other, furiously and freely. Daniel Tarantola, the Frenchman, and Peter Savage, an Englishman (now his close friend), disputed angrily. Each wrathful pair uttered their own equivalent of the time-honored phrase: "Care to step outside and say that again?" But the rest of the ritual never followed. The situation was defused by the very act of stepping outside and soon all was forgotten. Their sleep that night was the sweet sleep of exhausted warriors, secure in the knowledge of a famous victory.

At 10:30 on the morning of November 15, 1975, Stan Foster, Jason Weisfeld, Daniel Tarantola, and a few others were in the "submarine" at smallpox headquarters in Dacca. In quick succession three cables arrived: the first, from WHO in Geneva, read: *"Congratulations for Greatest Achievement."* The second, from the Center for Disease Control in Atlanta, read: *"Congratulations All Delighted."* The third was internal, and said: *"One suspected case smallpox detected Kuralia U.C South Dingaldi PS Bhola. Date of Detection 14/11/75. Date of Onset 30/10/75. Containment started, details to follow."*

Stunned though they all may have been, their reactions were totally professional. After the exhaustion of the final weeks, Dr. Jason Weisfeld, whose area included Bhola Island in the Ganges delta far away to the south, was poised to leave for a much needed vacation in Burma. He wanted to go straight back to Bhola, but Foster said no: "Jason, it is not – may not be – smallpox. You go off to Burma for your holiday." As the leader for the countrywide campaign, Foster took upon himself the responsibility to go down and verify the diagnosis.

First they had to determine just what credence one could put on the cable and how far back the contact had gone. (Subsequently, the date of onset of this case was identified as October 16, 1975, not October 30, as in the cable). Bhola Island had always been a problem: often the disease would not be reported, or only reported after an inordinate amount of time. The civil surgeon then had always been greatly embarrassed when smallpox was found in his province and so his smallpox officers had suppressed reports. Weisfeld says,

We had tried very hard to change that attitude, making it very clear that there was a positive good to come out of encouraging reporting rather than suppressing it. Nevertheless, I knew there were some officials who just wanted to see the zeros lined up on the reports from their various jurisdictions, who at times even took active measures to misclassify. If the sanitary inspector reported a rumor as chicken pox, or measles, they rarely bothered to verify the diagnosis, and failed to send doubtful specimens for laboratory investigation.

On the other hand there was an equally important consideration to be weighed in the balance. The cable had been sent by a team leader without the authority, or under the signatures, of any of the medical officials on the island. This man, Shahabudim, one of the very best fieldworkers around, was not a local person. He and his team, highly experienced and justifiably proud of their work, had recently been moved from Chittagong to Bhola Island. Shahabudim would never have notified Dacca until he was certain that the diagnosis had been confirmed and all proper procedures initiated.

If there was a single hero in this episode, it was Shahabudim. While the supervisors had been celebrating in Dacca, his team had continued working, checking outbreaks, investigating rumors, and going through the routines of doubt and belief. One morning they had stopped for a tea break and casually asked if anyone knew of any smallpox cases. An eleven-year-old girl, Bilkisunessa, who had herself recently recovered, mentioned that she thought she had seen a sick eight-year-old girl in the west of Bhola. When this girl was found she had fresh pox marks, so they knew that she had recently recovered. Tracing her contacts back along the human chain from one person to the next, the trail ended in the small village of Kuralia. There they found the patient whose existence prompted their cable. Ultimately they were to trace a whole chain of outbreaks in Bhola which had lain undetected for six months.

Stan Foster and one of his most capable fieldworkers, Alan Schnurr, left immediately. First they traveled down river on a paddle-wheeled steamer, the *Speedy Rocket,* taking twelve hours to get to Barisal that Sunday morning. From Barisal they went by speedboat to Bhola Island and landed only 200 meters from West Joynagar, the settlement that Bilkisunessa had pointed to as the source of infection. Then they took a Land Rover to Kuralia; once in the village they walked down a rough path to the hut that Shahabudim had identified.

As they walked, Schnurr's thoughts were in turmoil: "If we do find smallpox here," he worried, "what will be the impact on these people? And what is going to happen everywhere?" They walked down the pathway, and into the hut, and there in the corner, sticking out from under a pile of rags, they saw a tiny leg – covered with smallpox. Buried under the heap was a small three-year-old girl, Rahima Banu. As the strangers burst in, she screamed with fright. Quickly her mother picked her up and comforted her.

But just as quickly, Stan Foster, too, began to move. He appointed house guards and explained to the child's parents why no one could leave the house. The team started vaccinating that night, mobilizing everyone available on the island. They radioed headquarters and pulled into Bhola not only the best resident surveillance workers, but many people from other countries too.

Daniel Tarantola was in charge of the build-up. "It took us about three days to get organized after Stan's cable arrived. We hired a launch, called in five surveillance teams, and we went directly downstream." Two hundred people, with Land Rovers, motorbikes, outboard engines, fuel tanks, radios, bicycles, supplies, medicine, food, and vaccine, made up Tarantola's army. In a frenzy of sirens and activity, they pressed south as fast as they could. The trip took two days.

"Doing it this way was a calculated gamble," says Tarantola.

We were betting that there were no other cases in the country. If we'd been wrong it really would have been the end. Just one or two cases and the whole cycle would have restarted, for the monsoon was over and people were beginning to move round the country again. We'd been under tremendous pressure for a whole year to finish off the job. The government was losing patience and WHO was having problems finding continuing resources. But we were convinced that there were no more pockets of infection in the country so we pulled everyone onto the island.

A control headquarters was already set up in Bhola town by the time Tarantola arrived. Five guards, who provided a full twenty-four hours of constant cover, watched over the family and since no one was permitted to leave the house, food was provided. Then, village by village, house by house, the island of Bhola was systematically taken apart. During the first round, 100 percent of those living within a 1.5-mile radius of the infected house were vaccinated. A 5-mile radius was searched repeatedly by two teams: the first team did the work, the second assessed it, each looking continually for cases. The seven markets, nine schools, and local healers were frequently visited; every public place in every district – bus stations, ferries, *ghats*, crossroads – was checked again and again and again; all houses were repeatedly searched, each health worker covering twenty-five each day.

Bhola Island presented unique problems however. Reaching the outlying villages involved a difficult journey by bike or foot and the paths were regularly cut off by the tides. Yet searching these shore settlements was crucial, for they housed landless peasants, or fishermen, who wouldn't bother to report smallpox. So a launch, the *Madashi*, was commandeered and, in constant radio contact with headquarters, systematically covered every inlet, every creek, and every *char*.

Wide publicity accompanied the activity. Rewards of 580 *takas* ($1.50) were offered for verified reports and the message spread everywhere by posters, pamphlets, and handbills. The people were frightened, however. They hid smallpox because they believed that while those who reported would get money, those who were ill would have their houses burned. Rahima's great-uncle, Wazinddin, a man who had once had smallpox, was engaged as a public relations officer. He may have been unable to read or write, but he was superb as he exhorted, explained, and smoothed relations between the local people and the army of foreigners.

The first round of the island was completed in five days; the second, eight days later; 16,295 people of a total population of 18,150 were covered. Yet it was another two more months before everyone began to breathe easy. Normally they allowed six weeks to smother any given outbreak, but in this case they waited longer. One false announcement carried by the international press was quite enough and no one wanted to claim eradication prematurely for a second time, for the previous incident had precipitated a sizable reservoir of skepticism among the media and health professionals. As it was, *The New York Times* ran an article by Lawrence Altman under the headline "Smallpox Eradicated – Again!"

However, this time it was true: the last wild virus of *Variola major* had finally been extinguished. The campaign in Bangladesh had taken three years and eleven months, and had moved from a situation where, in 1971, 75 million people were cared for by three foreigners and twelve local people, to one where, in November 1975, one three-year-old girl was supported by 65 foreigners, 100 epidemiologists, 12,000 Bengali health workers, and a further 13,000 ancillary supporters.

Ironically Dr. Jason Weisfeld was also to be associated with the last naturally occurring case of the milder virus, *Variola minor*. He was in Somalia on October 26, 1976, when Ali Maow Maalin caught smallpox, and was ordered to stay for the duration of the case. Ali had contracted the disease while being helpful. Two people with active smallpox had been brought into Merkka by Land Rover but the driver couldn't find the isolation camp. He drove to the district hospital, but the sanitary inspector had gone home for lunch, so the hospital's medical officer ordered Ali, the hospital cook, to show the driver where the sanitary inspector lived. Ali got into the back of the Land Rover and sat next to two patients for less than five minutes – but that was enough. His smallpox was only diagnosed two weeks earlier, when he came down with a fever, but during those fourteen days, he'd made 120 contacts. These Jason Weisfeld had to find, vaccinate, and follow until he was certain that there were no further cases. Jason Weisfeld and Ali Maow Maalin still write to each other.

The whole world was now free of smallpox. The congratulations flooded in, and the reports and the articles came out, almost all, without exception, highly sanitized, dehumanized versions of this epic. Inevitably, postpartum depression set in and postmortems were set up. Most who took part were left with either permanent scars or permanent sensitivities and often both. Worse: smallpox had not yet finished with the human race. In England, the country where the successful weapon against the disease had been first tried, the final, Kafkaesque tragedy occurred. Two years later, the virus escaped from containment in research laboratories at Birmingham and killed Mrs. Janet Parker, a photographer who worked on the floor above. (Her mother also caught the disease but fortunately only mildly.) By 1978 only a few laboratories in the world were supposed to be holding the virus or any variety of it, and this laboratory at Birmingham was not among them. A week or so later Professor V. B. Bedson, a distinguished virologist and head of the research laboratory, slashed his wrists and died. Now the virus exists only in two WHO-inspected, high-security laboratories in Atlanta and Moscow, stored under the most secure conditions. All other laboratories in the world have destroyed their stocks.

It was some six years later that, in Europe, America, and Asia, I first met the scientists in this story; in the spring of 1984 we returned to Bangladesh to make a documentary film about their epic struggle. Nick Ward arrived from England, Stan Foster from Atlanta, Daniel Tarantola dropped in en route from Manila to a new assignment at WHO, and Lewis

Kaplan came in from Vanatua, the newly independent New Hebrides. Others, such as Karl Markvart and Geoffrey Taylor, were still in Dacca, never having left, and they and many Bangladeshis from all over the country, whether Ministry of Health bureaucrats or rural health workers, joined their friends in affectionate reminiscence.

The next few weeks took on the characteristics of a military reunion, when old-tried campaigners come together again. Exploits were recalled with pride, hardships with nostalgia, but, initially, with no real conviction. But as the days passed, in unprepared, unrehearsed moments, one by one, they revealed the depth of their experiences, relived some of the traumas, and echoed those aspects which they felt everyone should understand. The marvelous internationality was one constantly reiterated theme. People from twenty-two countries had been involved and the warm relationships that developed were among the most lasting features of the whole experience. Their closest friends come from those days and when they meet they move immediately to a level of warmth that they don't find in other relationships. Americans worked alongside Soviets, English alongside French, and years before the Camp David agreements were even considered, an Egyptian and an Israeli, jointly and happily, tackled one district in Bangladesh together, while each, unknown to the other, still continued to receive *Al-Ahrām* and the *Jerusalem Post* daily. And with mischievous humor, one foreigner in Bangladesh posted the local CIA man and the local KGB man to the same district. They got on famously, did an excellent job and, he suspects, when they weren't discussing smallpox, were probably talking shop.

Donald Henderson has his own special memories. "In 1966, when I went to Geneva, had I known what I learned by 1975 I would have said the whole task was impossible. But because we were all so ignorant, we grossly underestimated the problems, which actually turned out to be far worse than we ever imagined. And how wrong I was about the ending! The one country I believed would be quite impossible was Afghanistan."

Although Afghanistan's population was only twelve million, the health structure was appalling, for health teams never ventured into many areas, and cohorts of hereditary father-to-son variolators still moved across the country, with outbreak after outbreak of smallpox following them. Some tribal groups would not accept vaccination at all, and since most women were in purdah they could not be vaccinated by a male. Henderson went on,

When it came down to saying where would be the last case in the world, I was confident it would be Afghanistan. But two men and two women disproved my prediction. An Indian ex-colonel and a Pathan physician organized the program superbly, sending teams of vaccinators systematically through the countryside until they had made three complete circuits of Afghanistan. They even got to women in purdah by a mixture of carrot and stick, but no force was ever used. Had it been, they would have been shot. The two women – a Burmese nurse, four and a half feet tall, and a six-foot Russian – worked in the most remote areas and in impossible situations. The Russian was stoned and barely escaped with her life; the Burmese would travel on horseback with a gun over her shoulder – for decoration only, – which was both longer and taller than she. But they were brilliant, for they persuaded the government not to punish the variolators but instead invite them to use our vaccine instead of the traditional scabs. Such was the ingenuity of these four that smallpox was eradicated in Afghanistan two years before Asia was cleared.

In the intervening years however, Henderson has had to face many, and sometimes strident, criticisms as idealists battle with pragmatists about the methods used and the value of the end result. Some comments were present from the start and the most frequent spoke of aggressive teams of bulldozing foreigners, trampling all over WHO on the one hand and alien cultures on the other. Henderson commented:

You must realize that what you saw in Bangladesh was unique and very little that went on there occurred anywhere else. In the later stages of the campaign some "bulldozing" did become reality but this was definitely not so during most of its eleven-year duration. With three exceptions – Zaire, Afghanistan, and Nigeria – the number of international advisers assigned to any one country was usually no more than one or two people. But during the concluding phase, when the end appeared in sight and heroic measures seemed indicated, more foreigners were recruited – into India from 1973, into Bangladesh from 1974, into Ethiopia, and finally into Somalia in 1976.

There was a perfectly straightforward justification for this and for the methods employed. Everyone firmly believed the end truly *was* in sight, but they also recognized that should civil war erupt anywhere, the ultimate goal would be thwarted and the long-term results would be deleterious. These fears were not unfounded. You know now that the assassination of the president of Bangladesh in the summer of 1975 gave rise to a very real fear of another civil war there and shortly after this there was the terrible reality of the Somalia-Ethiopian war, whose outcome no one could predict.

Accordingly everyone worked flat out: nothing was postponed or omitted. Anything that could be done was done immediately, lest one neglected act might later be seen to be *the* one which allowed smallpox transmission to persist into a time when activities in the field were impossible. As things are presently, we couldn't do it now. There'd be no way to get into Afghanistan or Iran, for a start. So the aggressive approach was characteristic of only one short period in the program and occurred in only a few countries.

This is not to say that the bureaucratic procedures were not circumvented at times. You have seen that they were. But for the most part, and for most of the years in most of the countries, it was not only necessary but *mandatory* to work within the constraints of the local political systems. These were less than perfect but quite adequate to get the job done. And I am personally convinced that the same end result could eventually have been achieved in Bangladesh, Somalia, and Ethiopia, by the same methods and at the same pace as in all other countries. But it would have required several more years, and unfortunately these were the years when no one knew whether work would be possible because of likely civil disorders.

Donald Henderson's assessment and reservations are echoed by those people whose experiences were entirely in the last countries to report smallpox. Some of them are still concerned that their heroic efforts might, in part, have been counterproductive. For the rapid importation of international advisers did not permit the slow build-up of national staffs such as took place in many other countries, and they are regretful that this was inevitably so.

"There were real defects to our program," admitted Stan Foster. "We had money and enthusiasm, but it was not a developmental effort and we were forced into doing things we couldn't sustain."

"The military aspect of the campaign worried us a lot," said Nick Ward in his turn.

We had a target and we went for it. I suppose you could say that we cared more about our objective than the people we were there to help. But on the other hand, our campaign demonstrated something very important – something that people said could not be done. It showed that we could eradicate a disease in a poor country in spite of inadequate health services. Provided one can mobilize the inherent creative energy of a people, then anything is possible. And that's really all we did: we were just the catalysts.

"We also have to remember how good WHO turned out to be," echoed Tarantola. "As an international institution it may have its defects, but it's one of the best humanity has ever created. They changed their usual routines for this campaign and worked directly through people rather than through governments, and got quite used to long-haired, pony-tailed workers in T-shirts, periodically showing up in their corridors."

Some people assert flatly, however, that the rationale for eradication was based on Western values. Smallpox represented a natural process that should *not* have been interfered with. People were fatalistic about the disease since they had known it for centuries, and knowing death from many causes, had secure constructs to cope. Moreover, compared with cholera or malaria, it was minor and unimportant and thus, these idealists argue, not only was the objective misguided but irrelevant: Western ideas of health were imposed on these societies. Those who worked in the campaign reject this argument with scorn. Nick Ward is one: "Such attitudes ignore those individuals who suffered. Smallpox was always a disease of the poor in the *bastis* and the ghettos. Wealthy people and their children were mostly vaccinated. Those who saw, or who felt, or who smelled, the distress the disease could cause – who realized the impact of blindness on an individual and their family – could never hold such views."

The same critics argue that the campaign is a bad model for the future for it cost so much that its success gives the impression that cash conquers all problems. But, first, while the campaign might have seemed enormously expensive, it was actually very cheap. For developed countries the cost was trivial, certainly when compared with current military expenditures or even with the cost of vaccinating travelers and containing epidemics. The total sum involved for the entire eleven years was $300 million; of this, over one-third ($120 million) came from the endemic countries themselves, whether in cash or kind. Second, no one can seriously believe that cash conquers all problems. It helps certainly, but, still the campaign would have failed without personal relationships, which cannot be bought.

The campaign's success achieved a number of very important ends over and above the eradication of a disease. It gave an enormous boost to people in charge of health within the developing countries, where the status of the ministries of health is usually very low. It also gave resident health workers a new confidence and motivation, as well as making a huge contribution to their society's understanding of disease control. The success of the smallpox campaign subtly changed the attitudes in their communities: things are *not* irrevocably written; people *can* determine their fate; the spring still comes every year but smallpox does not. So eradicating smallpox has created a demand from people for other health programs and, in the end, their governments will have to listen.

There are two final, important points. The people in this continuing saga altered the course of human history for the better, and the world will never be the same again. The episodes in the campaign show the tapestry of human endeavor at its best, and even in those parts some may find questionable, there was nothing that approaches the degradation or sheer barbarity that we see each day in the world around us. Moreover, this epic illustrates something for which, for once, the human race may be gloriously proud. Happily, René Dubos's fears turned out to be totally unfounded. He had predicted that failure would depend totally on people and relationships between them – but these turned out to be superb. In the history of the world, whenever before have we ever cooperated together like this to achieve such a glorious end?

So the story had a happy ending as all best stories should. But what is a happy ending? What does the eradication of smallpox mean to the mass of the rural poor in Bangladesh? What does it mean to Rahima Banu and her family?

Rahima, now twelve, is the eldest of four. One after the other her three younger brothers arrived in quick succession. Thin and malnourished, she will never gain normal childhood growth, and over a few years her father watched helplessly as flood waters washed away the five acres he possessed. Landless, he was forced to take casual labor as a fisherman, earning one-eighth of the catch – if a catch were caught – an amount quite insufficient to feed his family. With the small amount of money that came when Rahima was identified as the last person in the world to have *Variola major*, he bought half an acre but had to borow money from a money lender, at extortionate interest, to build a house (a roof supported by pillars but with no walls). By now, he was heavily in debt. A quick collection from all of us discharged this debt and there was enough money left over to buy two cows. But over the years, the spiral of poverty has dragged him and his family down, not through indolence on his part, but through the sheer surge of circumstance. His story is typical of millions in the developing world.

On the one hand it was deeply moving, even romantic, to talk to this girl who represents the last link in a human chain along which the smallpox virus passed for generations in history as far back as the Egyptian king, Ramses V, 1,160 B.C. However, there was not one shred of romance to realize that so bad are their circumstances that its eradication was just a minor thing for this family; it meant no more spring disease. But there is so much else to contend with: the continuing spiral of poverty, malnutrition, and our indifference. We cannot pontificate, or advise others about what steps they should take with family planning and the like, for we must realize that these people cannot even conceive a future for *themselves*, let alone their children. All they can do is to struggle as best they can, minute by minute, day by day. Though we can take a great deal of pride in the episode just recorded, we, the rich, have still done only one very small thing for them, the poor.

———————————

Finally, at the end of our time in Bangladesh, I challenged my friends: "Face it," I said. "You're all talking with great nostalgia but when the end came you were thankful to be leaving."

The replies were unanimous. "We were deeply thankful. Matters had gone on too long and if we hadn't been successful in 1975 we never would have been. We couldn't have taken another year."

But already they have taken up the next challenge. Since humanity is the thing these doctors cherish most, they will always walk directly toward humanity's problems, working to save lives and giving the whole of their lives to do so. Thus many of the members of the Order of the Bifurcated Needle are gearing up for the next major international health initiative and will soon be hard at work in remote places as far apart as the New Hebrides, Colombia, and Senegal. Underwritten by WHO, UNICEF, the Rockefeller Foundation, the World Bank, and the United Nations' Development Program, a comprehensive global immunization scheme for children is under way when, everywhere, routine shots against measles, mumps, tuberculosis, diphtheria, tetanus, polio, whooping cough, and probably hepatitis B too, will be offered in the way we take for granted in Western society. Known as the children's revolution, this is the only revolution I unreservedly support. The program has learned from the smallpox experience: its executants rely on local people, build on and extend local infrastructures so doing immunization within the context of primary health care. Maternal and general health education will be added too, and finally family planning. Older and wiser, but enthusiastic as ever, their eyes firmly fixed on their new lodestar, realizing that as before, success will depend a great deal on Donald Henderson's and Bill Foege's capacity to inspire cohorts of people; many members of the Order of the Bifurcated Needle have already started work.

But they do still have one small loose end of their own to tie up. For on more than one occasion Henderson made a promise to all those who were working for him, one he would fulfill, he said, when smallpox was eradicated. Of all the thousands of promises he made, in the ten years, nine months, and twenty-six days of the global campaign, this was the only one he did not keep. So one day they are all going down to Johns Hopkins University in Baltimore and together they will march into the office of the dean of the School of Public Health and in unison, they will announce: "D. A., we've come to watch you smoke your last cigarette."

Series Acknowledgments

Script by
Michael Latham and June Goodfield (The Kuru Mystery, Vaccine on Trial, The Three Valleys
of St. Lucia, The Last Wild Virus)
David Collison and June Goodfield
(The Last Outcasts), based on
the book *Quest for the Killers*
by June Goodfield.

A Production of Video Arts Television, London, and WGBH Boston
in association with Channel 4, U.K.

Copyright 1985 by Dumbarton
Films Ltd. and WGBH Educational
Foundation

Series Producer
Michael Latham

Producer for WGBH-TV
Jo Elwyn-Jones

Associate Producer
  (The Kuru Mystery)
Michael Johnstone

Film Editors
Brenda Taylor
  (Vaccine on Trial)
Beryl Wilkins
  (The Three Valleys of St. Lucia)
Gregory Harris
  (The Last Outcasts)
Fiona Gillespie
  (The Last Wild Virus)

Directors
Jim Black (The Kuru Mystery)
Mike Gibbon (Vaccine on Trial)
Michael Houldey
  (The Three Valleys of St. Lucia)
David Collison
  (The Last Outcasts)
Alan Patient (The Last Wild Virus)

WGBH and the publisher wish to
thank

Ciba-Geigy Corporation

Merck & Co., Inc.

Pfizer Inc.

Squibb Corporation

who sponsored the television series
based on this book.

Other Books by June Goodfield

Courier to Peking, 1973

The Siege of Cancer, 1975

*Playing God: Genetic Engineering
and the Manipulation of Life,* 1977

*Reflections on Science and the
Media,** 1981

*An Imagined World: A Study of
Scientific Creativity,* 1981

**Wissenchaft und Medien,* 1983
German-language edition,
        Birkhäuser, Basel

Quest for the Killers

Copy edited by Cynthia I. Benn
Designed by Jack Foley
Composed by DEKR Corporation
      in Sabon
Printed by Alpine Press Inc.
      on 70 lb. Stora Matte
Bound by Alpine Press Inc.
      in Holliston Mills Roxite B
Color insert and cover printed by
      New England Book Components
      on 80 lb. C2S Warrenflo